AAS 6
Agents and Actions Supplements

Prostaglandins and Inflammation:

Conference, London, 1979

held at King's College Hospital Medical School,
University of London, Denmark Hill, London, on
2nd – 3rd August, 1979.

Edited by K. D. Rainsford and A. W. Ford-Hutchinson.

Birkhäuser Verlag
Basel · Boston · Stuttgart

Edited by:
K. D. Rainsford, Biochemistry Department, University of
Tasmania, Hobart, Tasmania, Australia
and
A. W. Ford-Hutchinson, Biochemical Pharmacology Research Group,
King's College Hospital Medical School, University of London,
Denmark Hill, London, England.

This international Conference was held at Normanby College,
King's College Hospital, Denmark Hill, London, on 2nd and 3rd
August 1979 to enable a critical evaluation of the role of
prostaglandins in inflammation and related aspects.

Library of Congress Cataloging in Publication Data

Symposium on Prostaglandins and Inflammation,
    King's College Hospital Medical School, 1979.
    Proceedings of the Symposium on Prostaglandins
and Inflammation.
    (Agents and actions: supplements; 6)
    1. Inflammation – Congresses. 2. Prostaglandins
– Congresses. I. Rainsford, K. D., 1941 –
II. Ford-Hutchinson, A. W.
IV. Series. [DNLM: 1. Inflammation – Immunity –
Congresses. 2. Prostaglandins – Pharmacodynamics –
Congresses. 3. Anti-inflammatory agents –
Pharmacodynamics – Congresses. 4. Inflammation –
Physiopathology – Congresses. WI AG33A v. 6 /
QW700 S9894p 1977]
RB131. S97 1979   616'.047   79–22502
ISBN-13: 978-3-0348-7234-8   e-ISBN-13: 978-3-0348-7232-4
DOI: 10.1007/978-3-0348-7232-4

CIP-Kurztitelaufnahme der Deutschen Bibliothek

Prostaglandins and inflammation: conference, London,
1979, held at King's College Hospital Med. School,
Univ. of London, London, on 2.–3. August 1979 / ed.
by K. D. Rainsford and A. W. Ford-Hutchinson. –
Basel, Boston, Stuttgart: Birkhäuser, 1979.
    (Agents and actions: Suppl.; 6)
    ISBN-13: 978-3-0348-7234-8
NE: Rainsford, Kay D. [Hrsg.]; Medical School <London,
King's College>

TABLE OF CONTENTS

Preface

Since prostaglandins were first proposed as mediators of inflammation some eight years ago, there have been a variety of arachidonic acid metabolites discovered including the thromboxanes, prostacyclin, prostaglandin endoperoxides and lipoxygenase products such as SRS-A. All of them have subsequently been shown to have significant and specific biological activities not only in inflammatory responses but also in other physiological processes. The explosion of research in this area has been an indication of the importance of this field but has also meant that it is time for an evaluation of activities of prostaglandins and products of the arachidonate pathway - collectively described as eicosanoids. For this reason the organizers of this conference felt it was timely to bring together workers in the field and critically evaluate some aspects of the role of different eicosanoids in inflammatory responses and the action of the anti-inflammatory agents drugs used to modulate or inhibit these responses.

The conference held at King's College Hospital Medical School produced lively and constructive discussions. While there are still many complexities to be investigated several important conclusions did emerge. The organizers were grateful to have the use of facilities at Normanby College and King's College Hospital. Also we would like to thank the Boots Company Ltd., for generous sponsorship and Mrs. P. Carter for valuable secretarial assistance.

K. D. Rainsford
A. W. Ford-Hutchinson
M. J. H. Smith

Organizers.

INTRODUCTION TO PROSTAGLANDINS AND INFLAMMATION

G. P. Lewis
Royal College of Surgeons of England

        As an introduction I thought it might be useful for
me to point out some of the most recent advances which will
be discussed in more detail by various contributors and
perhaps refer to some of the gaps which still have to be
filled.
        First, we are going to hear about the pathways of
arachidonic acid metabolism from Bob Jones.   Immediately I
am in a difficulty because I have already been told that I
cannot show any slides about pathways because Dr. Jones is
going to show them all.   In spite of that I have no doubt
that we shall see several versions of the pathways from
arachidonic acid during the next two days.
        However, in addition to these, there are some
important pathways before arachidonic acid with which I
thought I should start off.   It still seems most likely, as
pointed out by Walter Vogt and his colleagues, that the main
source of arachidonic acid is a membrane phospholipid.   On
the other hand, it has been established that in certain
situations there are alternate sources of arachidonic acid,
such as neutral lipids or triglycerides (1,2).   This
particular source becomes relatively more important in
tissues which contain a high proportion of neutral lipids
such as adipose tissue.   Furthermore, cholesterol esters
which are often deposited in blood vessels are also capable
of providing arachidonic acid.   These esters contain a high

proportion of linoleic acid which can be readily converted
to arachidonic acid via the ubiquitous acetyl-CoA system.
These alternate sources of arachidonate are important when we
come to consider inhibition of the prostaglandin (PG) system
by compounds, the action of which results in the inhibition
of phospholipase A_2.

      The pathways which lead from arachidonic acid will
be covered very comprehensively by Dr. Jones but I must
mention the exciting new discovery of Bengt Samuelsson and
his colleagues (4th International Prostaglandin Conference,
1979). They have made the first proposal for the complete
structure of an SRS. It has been clear for some time that the
elusive mediator SRS-A was closely associated with the
lipoxygenase pathways of arachidonic acid metabolism.
Priscilla Piper, in my own department, together with Howard
Morris from Imperial College have been very close in the
hunt for the structure of SRS-A and we shall hear from Dr.
Morris about this work. It looks as if most of their findings agree with Samuelsson's view of the structure. A few
years ago it certainly would have been difficult to imagine
SRS-A to be a triene metabolite of arachidonic acid combined
with a molecule of cysteine; but now that we have the
structure and the possibility of specific antagonists, there
is almost certain to be an explosion of research in this
part of the metabolic pathways of arachidonic acid.

      The next section of our meeting deals with PGs as
mediators of acute inflammation. I think in the area of
the vascular effects of PGs in inflammation we have a most
important developing theory. This is the two-mediator
theory developed mainly by Tim Williams in my department (3).
I am going to take a little time to discuss it because,
although John Westwick will no doubt mention the work, I
imagine that he will concentrate more on the relative
activities of the PGs as vasodilators.

      We have previously thought of mediators of acute
inflammation as endogenous substances which account for all
or many of the cardinal signs of inflammation. So with
bradykinin, for instance, we tried to persuade everybody
that it was potent in producing vasodilatation, increasing
vascular permeability, inducing pain and even causing
migration of polymorphonuclearleucocytes (PMNs). Dr.
Williams's idea is that in order to produce a large increase

in plasma exudation which one sees in inflammation, two
actions are necessary - vasodilatation and increased vascular
permeability.   He has suggested that these effects are
produced by different mediators and has illustrated this in
rabbit skin measuring blood flow by a ^{133}Xe clearance
technique and plasma exudation by the extravasation of ^{131}I-
albumin.   In rabbit skin, bradykinin causes an increase in
vascular permeability but not a maximal increase in blood
flow.   The result is a small amount of plasma exudation.
Prostaglandins E_2 or I_2 are very potent vasodilators, but
hardly affect vascular permeability - the result is little
or no plasma exudation.   When the two are injected together
there is a marked plasma exudation, because bradykinin is
increasing the permeability and the PG increasing blood flow.
        The second point that he has shown is that such a
combination of effects occurs in inflammatory reactions in
vivo.   Using injections of pertussis vaccine (4) or together
with Sanaa Kenawy and myself (5) using the Arthus reaction, it
was possible to show that the significant plasma exudation
which occurred in the reaction could be accounted for in this
way.   Indomethacin reduces the plasma exudation in these
reactions although we know that PGs do not increase vascular
permeability.   However, if PGE_2 or I_2 are injected into the
reaction site in the presence of indomethacin, the plasma
exudation is again evident.   This means that in the presence
of indomethacin, there is present an endogenous substance
which increases vascular permeability, but does not by itself
cause an increase in plasma exudation.   Using anti-histamines
and inhibitors of bradykinin formation, it was not possible
to affect the plasma exudation indicating that the agent was
not histamine or bradykinin.   So in this indirect way, i.e.
using it in combination with a PG, it has been possible to
demonstrate the existence of an unknown agent which increases
vascular permeability.   Tim Williams and Peter Jose have
gone further than this, but I do not feel justified in saying
more on their behalf at present.
        It is known that the pain produced by bradykinin or
histamine is also potentiated by prostaglandins.   Whether
this is the result of the vasodilatation they produce, is not
clear, but perhaps we will find out from Dr. Tyers.
        This afternoon we shall have two talks on pyrexia.
It seemed to me that Feldberg (6) did such a good job on PGs
and pyrexia that I wonder what else can be said.   He observed

that PG levels in cerebro-spinal fluid changed in direct
proportion with pyrogenic fever.   When the fever was reduced
with aspirin, so the PG levels were reduced.   Perhaps
inflammation-pyrexia is somewhat different and we shall have
Dr. Cranston to tell us about that.

The two cells that may take part in acute inflammation that are going to be discussed by our host Mervyn Smith
and Dr. Chignard in the following session, are PMNs and
platelets. PMNs have long been known to be one of the first
cells to appear at the site of an acute inflammatory reaction.
It has never been absolutely clear to me what they are
supposed to do - phagocytose offending organisms or materials,
or secrete lytic enzyme systems, or take up immune complexes.
Now we might ask - do they carry to the site of inflammation
substances which we normally regard as endogenous mediators
such as PGs or the enzymes or substrates which give rise to
them? Furthermore, do they carry soluble substances which
interact with other cells? For example, are the PMNs the
first line cells responsible for the recruitment of the
monocytes which appear later?

As for platelets, there has been an enormous amount
of work done on platelets in relation to the PG system.
Their aggregation by thromboxane and inhibition of the reaction
by prostacyclin has been a fascinating story. But the role
that platelets play in inflammatory reactions, is a mystery -
but perhaps we might be presented with some of the answers
today. The possibility that platelets with the unique
thromboxane-synthetase system play a role in inflammation
raises some difficult questions. Do they give rise to
thromboxane at the site of inflammation, and if so, what does
it do? Does it cause further platelet aggregation or
produce vasoconstriction, or exert some as yet unknown action?
I think that here is an example of the need for care in
considering different types of inflammation as different
entities and not regarding them all as identical reactions.
Perhaps it is in the type of inflammation where there is
serious vascular damage that platelets are called upon to
play a role.

The second morning of this meeting is devoted to
PGs in chronic inflammation and is introduced by Ivan Bonta.
John Morley and Philip Davies are going to discuss the
possibilities of PGs acting as soluble mediators of cell-cell
interactions.   Dr. Morley and his colleagues worked out a

very interesting picture of the etiology of rheumatoid
arthritis based on the PG system.   The macrophages are
activated by a lymphokine secreted by sensitised lymphocytes.
The activated macrophages produce a PG which inhibits the
sensitised lymphocytes from secreting more lymphokines (7).
It was suggested that this was a normal negative feed-back
mechanism which controlled the activity of lymphocytes.   It
was also suggested that if rheumatoid subjects had an inborn
fault such as the lack of reactivity to E-type PGs by the
lymphocytes, then lymphocyte activities would go unchecked
leading to a chronic disorder (8).   I hope we will be
informed of the development of this hypothesis as well as   the
latest results about this important area of mediators of cell-
cell interactions.   But let us not forget that there are
other important mediators of such effects.   Dudley Dumonde
and his colleagues (9) have carried out a lot of work on the
action of lymphokines as mediators of cellular activities
and David Gordon and I are starting some work on the influence
of histamine on cell-cell interactions.   We must be careful
that whilst paying adequate attention to the PGs, we must not
be overcome by their importance to the extent of believing
that they account for all the important features of
inflammation.
        Friday morning will be wound up by further discuss-
ions on PGs and macrophages from Tony Ford Hutchinson of the
host department and K. Brune .   I hope that by the end of
these sessions we might know which type of PG is formed by
macrophages and whether their function is related to vascular
changes or to cell-cell interactions.
        The organisers of this meeting were quite relentless
in their planning.   Rather than having the meeting gradually
tail off during Friday afternoon, they have packed the afternoon with contributions on two very important areas of
research.   The first is the effect of anti-inflammatory drugs
on the PG system and the second is an attempt to answer the
question - are the side-effects of anti-inflammatory agents
due to their effect on the PG system.
        On the first of these topics I shall be very
interested to hear of any serious argument against the view
that aspirin-like anti-inflammatory drugs exert their
vascular and analgesic actions by inhibition of PG synthesis.
It seems to me that the case for this view has grown stronger

over the years.   Furthermore, it appears that their main
toxic side-effects on the gastro-intestinal tract and possibly
that on the kidney result from their effect on the PG system.
It would be extremely helpful if, during these last two
sessions, we could have some strong views on these points.
It is important because we want to know whether we should
look for anti-inflammatory drugs which inhibit PG synthetase.
If the answer is 'yes' then should we use such a simple test
as a primary screen for new anti-inflammatory drugs.   If the
answer is 'no' then should we avoid the property of inhibiting
cyclo-oxygenase in a new anti-inflammatory drug in an attempt
to produce an agent without the usual side-effects.
        There is one other aspect of this particular
problem.   Is there some differential specificity of the
cyclo-oxygenases in different tissues?   There was a
suggestion some years ago that such specificity existed but
this work does not appear to have been followed up.   I should
like to know if it is possible to develop drugs which inhibit
the cyclo-oxygenase producing PGs at a site of inflammation
without interfering with the PGs which maintain the vascular
integrity   of areas like the gastric mucosa.
        There is a further complication as a result of the
discovery of the pathways of arachidonic acid metabolism
leading to thromboxane and prostacyclin.   Compounds are
being developed which specifically inhibit thromboxane or
prostacyclin synthetase without inhibiting cyclo-oxygenase.
This leads us to the question - will such compounds be
effective in any type of inflammatory reaction and could the
inhibition of such specific pathways avoid toxic side-effects?
        One final area of interest which does not appear in
the programme is the effect of glucocorticoids on the PG
system.   As some of you know, this is one of my own personal
interests, so I would just like to finish this introduction
with a few words about the present state of our knowledge in
this area.   When we first examined the action of glucocorticoids on the PG system in adipose tissue, we found that
the release of PGs was inhibited but that some synthesis still
continued in the tissue although this could still be inhibited
by indomethacin (10).   We thought at first that this was an
effect on the membranes of the fat cells.   However,
Gryglewski and his colleagues (11) showed that steroids
inhibited not only the release of PGs but also the release of

arachidonic acid from lung tissue.   Later, we could confirm
this inhibition of arachidonic acid release from adipose
tissue.   Furthermore, we showed in fat cell ghosts that
while the steroids inhibited the release of arachidonic acid
from the membrane phospholipids, they potentiated its release
from the neutral lipids (12).   We must assume, therefore,
that the PG synthesis which continues in the presence of
glucocorticoids originates from the arachidonic acid present
in the neutral lipids.   Of course, in adipose tissue this
is a very significant fraction which is probably why we
were able to make the observation in the first place.

Pursuing our earlier speculation, we have examined
in more detail the action of drugs including steroids on
membranes using multi-bilayer liposomes made of dipalmitoyl
lecithin (13).   Although drugs like cholesterol and some
anaesthetics can alter the membrane fluidity and thereby the
activity of membrane-bound enzymes by interacting with the
phospholipids of the membrane, we could find no evidence of
interaction between glucocorticoids and the phospholipids.
Furthermore, using the liposomes in combination with purified
phospholipase A_2 and measuring hydrolysis spectrophotometric-
ally we could not detect any evidence of a direct action of
the glucocorticoids on the enzyme itself.

One more piece of evidence against the interaction
of steroids with cell membrane was provided by an experiment
using fat cell ghosts.   When labelled PG was incorporated
inside the ghost during their preparation, it was possible to
measure its leakage.   The first interesting point was that
the cell membrane was very resistant to the passage of PG
and about 70% of the labelled $PGF_2\alpha$ remained inside the cell
after incubation for 2 hours.   Secondly, the presence of
glucocorticoids, hydrocortisone or dexamethasone did not
affect this slow leakage which indicates that the steroids
do not act on the membrane as we originally suspected.
However, the fact that the PGs passed through the cell
membranes so slowly seems to indicate that they are not
generally formed inside cells.   One is tempted to suggest
that PG formation in fat cells and perhaps in other cells too,
may go on primarily in the membrane, in which case its
release would not be inhibited by the impermeability of
the cell membrane.

We have, therefore, to look for an alternative site of action of glucocorticoids. Most recently, we have been examining their effect on cAMP with the consequent re-distribution of intracellular calcium. However, some others have suggested that the action of steroids required RNA and protein synthesis (14) while a further suggestion is that the glucocorticoids initiate the synthesis of an inhibitor of phospholipase A_2 (15). No doubt we shall hear about this at future meetings.

Meanwhile, during the next two days I have no doubt that much more detail will be revealed in those areas under discussion. I have tried to pose as many relevant questions as possible. Let us hope that when it comes to summing up we shall have more exclamation marks than question marks.

REFERENCES

1.   Lewis, G.P. and Piper, P.J. Biochem.Pharmacol., 27, 1409-1412 (1978)

2.   Christ, E.J. and Nugteren, D.H. Biochim.biophys.Acta, 218, 296-307 (1970)

3.   Williams, T.J. Br. J. Pharmac., 65, 517-524 (1979)

4.   Williams, T.J. and Peck M.J. Nature, 270. 530-532, (1977)

5.   Kenawy, S., Lewis. G.P. and Williams, T.J. 7th Int. Congr.Pharmacol. Paris. (1978)

6.   Feldberg, W. In: The role of prostaglandins in inflammation. (Ed.G.P. Lewis) pp47-56, (1976) Bern: Huber.

7.   Gordon, D., Bray, M.A. and Morley, J. Nature, 262, 401-402 (1976)

8.   Morley, J. Prostaglandins, 8, 315-326 (1974)

9.   Dumonde, D.C. Ann. Immunol., 2, 129. (1970)

10. Lewis, G.P. and Piper, P.J. Nature, 254, 308-311 (1975)

11. Gryglewski, R.J., Bogumila, P., Korbut, R., Grodzinska,L. and Ocetkiewicz. A. Prostaglandins, 10, 343-355 (1975)

12.   Lewis, G.P., Piper, P.J. and Vigo, C. Br.J.Pharmac.,
      (1979) in press.

13.   Vigo, C., Lewis, G.P. and Piper, P.J. Biochem.Pharmacol.,
      (1979) in press

14.   Danon, A. and Assouline, G. Nature, 273, 552-554 (1978)

15.   Flower, R.J. and Blackwell, G.J. Nature, 278, 456-459
      (1979)

Chapter One

METABOLISM OF ARACHIDONIC ACID

PATHWAYS OF ARACHIDONIC ACID METABOLISM

R.L. Jones
Department of Pharmacology, University of Edinburgh.

        Unsaturated fatty acids are susceptible to both
chemical and enzymic oxidation processes involving the utilisa-
tion of molecular oxygen.   Chemical attack may occur either by
autoxidation where the lipid catalyses its own oxidation or
through catalysis by haematin compounds, the latter but not the
former being inhibited by cyanide.   A widely studied enzymic
peroxidation is that catalysed by soya bean lipoxygenase (1).
Linoleic acid is attacked by the enzyme at two positions C9 and
C13, to yield respectively 9D-hydroperoxy-octadeca-10 trans, 12
cis-dienoic acid and 13L-hydroperoxy-octadeca-9 cis, 11 trans-
dienoic acid.   Several iso-enzymes of the soya bean lipoxygenase
have been isolated, differing in the relative amounts of the 9-
and 13- hydroperoxides produced, pH optima, and rates of reaction
with linoleate, methyl linoleate and trilinolein (2,3).   Lip-
oxygenase-1 rapidly forms 15-hydroperoxyeicosa-5 cis, 8 cis, 11
cis, 13 trans-tetraenoic acid from arachidonic acid (4,5,6)
(Fig.1).   Further oxygenation occurs more slowly at the C8
position to produce a dihydroperoxy compound (7).   In contrast
lipoxygenase-2 produces considerable amounts of a trihydroxy-
furan from arachidonic acid (Fig.2) (8).   This substance is
apparently identical to that isolated and characterised from
incubation of arachidonic acid with sheep seminal vesicles by
Pace-Asciak (9).

        Only recently have similar lipoxygenase enzymes been
characterised in animal tissues.   Hamberg and Samuelsson (10)
and Nugteren (11) reported the presence of a lipoxygenase in
blood platelets which converts arachidonic acid into 12-hydro-
peroxy-eicosa-5 cis, 8 cis, 10 trans, 14 cis-tetraenoic acid
(12-HPETE) (Fig.3).   The initially formed hydroperoxide may
undergo a number of further transformations and the reader is
referred to papers by Hamberg (12) and Gardner (13) on the
decomposition of linoleic acid hydroperoxides.

        In the case of 12-HPETE reduction to the 12-hydroxy
acid readily occurs.   Several other products found on incubation of human platelets with arachidonic acid may also derive
from 12-HPETE.   The 11,12-epoxy-10-hydroxy-eicosatrienoic acid
shown in Fig.3 has been isolated as two isomeric forms;   the

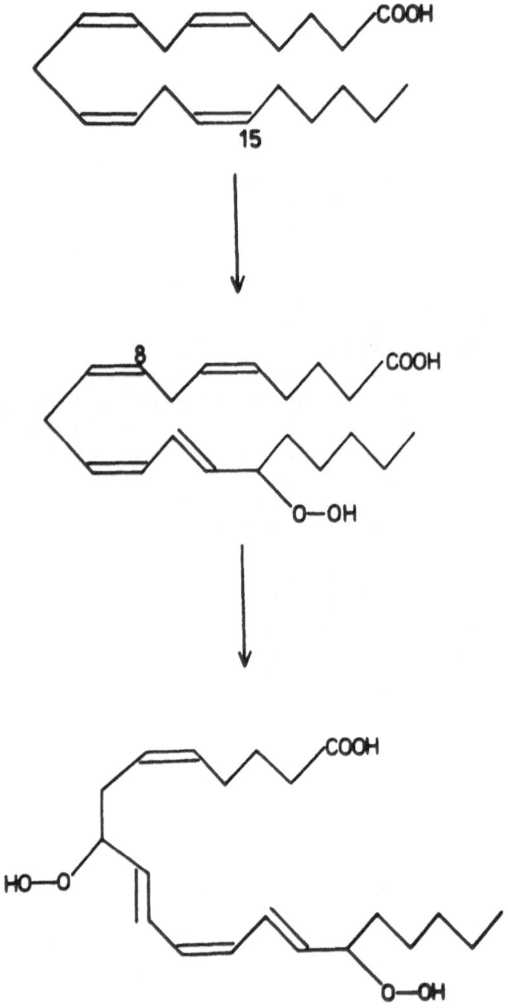

<u>Fig. 1</u>

Reaction of soya bean lipoxygenase-1 with arachidonic acid.

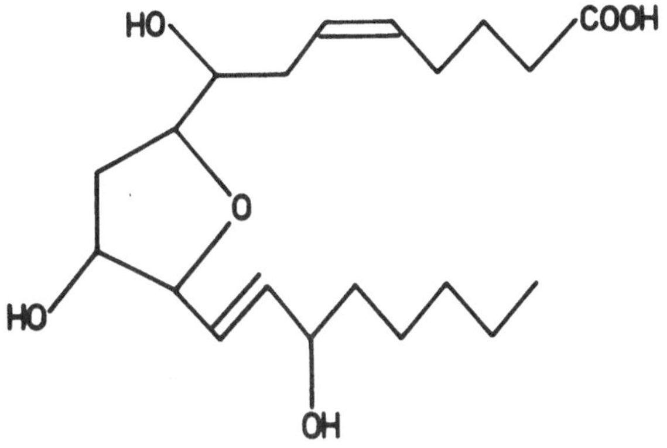

<u>Fig. 2</u>

        Proposed structure of a trihydroxy-furan derived
from reaction of arachidonic acid with soya bean lipoxygenase-2
and subsequent treatment with sodium dithionite.

corresponding 10,11,12-trihydroxy hydration product was not
found.   The more polar of the epoxides showed chemotactic
activity for rabbit peritoneal leucocytes (14);   similar
activity has been reported for 12-HETE (15).   Two trihydroxy
acids, 8,11,12-THETA and 8,9,12-THETA, were also present in the
platelet extract but the postulated 11,12-epoxy-8-hydroxy
intermediate could not be identified (16,17) (Fig.3).   This
difference probably reflects the greater resistance to hydration
of the non-allylic epoxide compared to the allylic epoxide.

        Samuelsson and co-workers (18) have shown that hydro-
peroxy insertion can also occur at C5 in the arachidonic acid
molecule (Fig.4).   The hydroperoxide undergoes a further
transformation with overall loss of a molecule of water to give

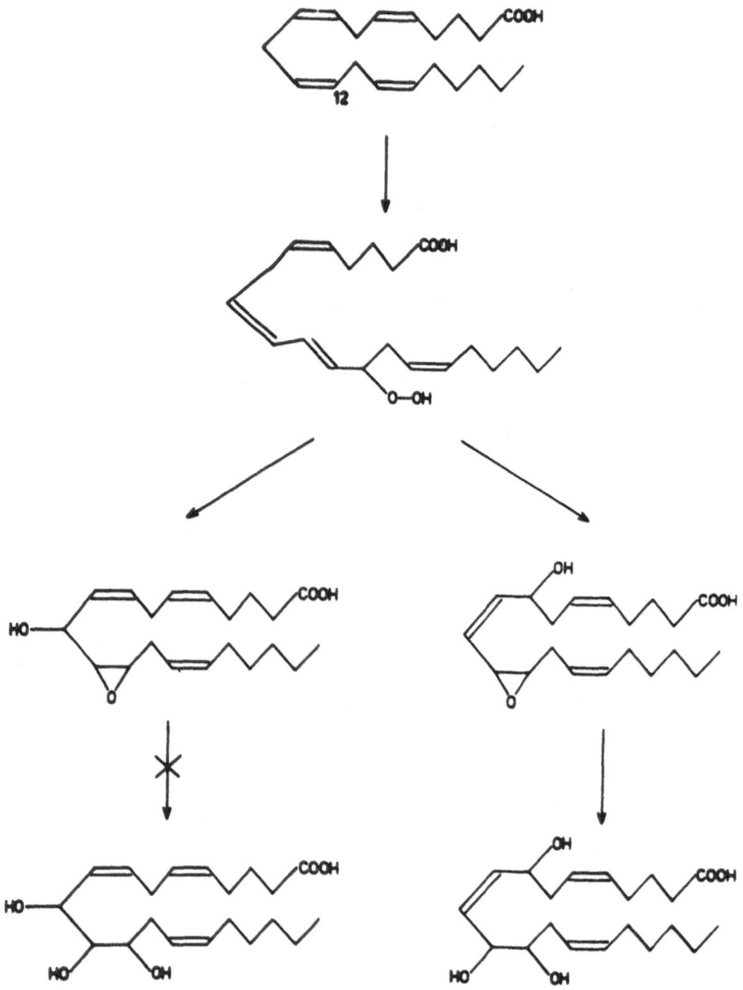

Fig. 3

Production of 12-HPETE from arachidonic acid and
possible further transformations. The lower right compound is
3,11,12-trihydroxy-eicosa-5,9,14-trienoic acid (8,11,12-THETA)
and is always found with the isomeric 8,9,12-trihydroxy-
eicosa-5,11,14-trienoic acid (8,9,12-THETA).

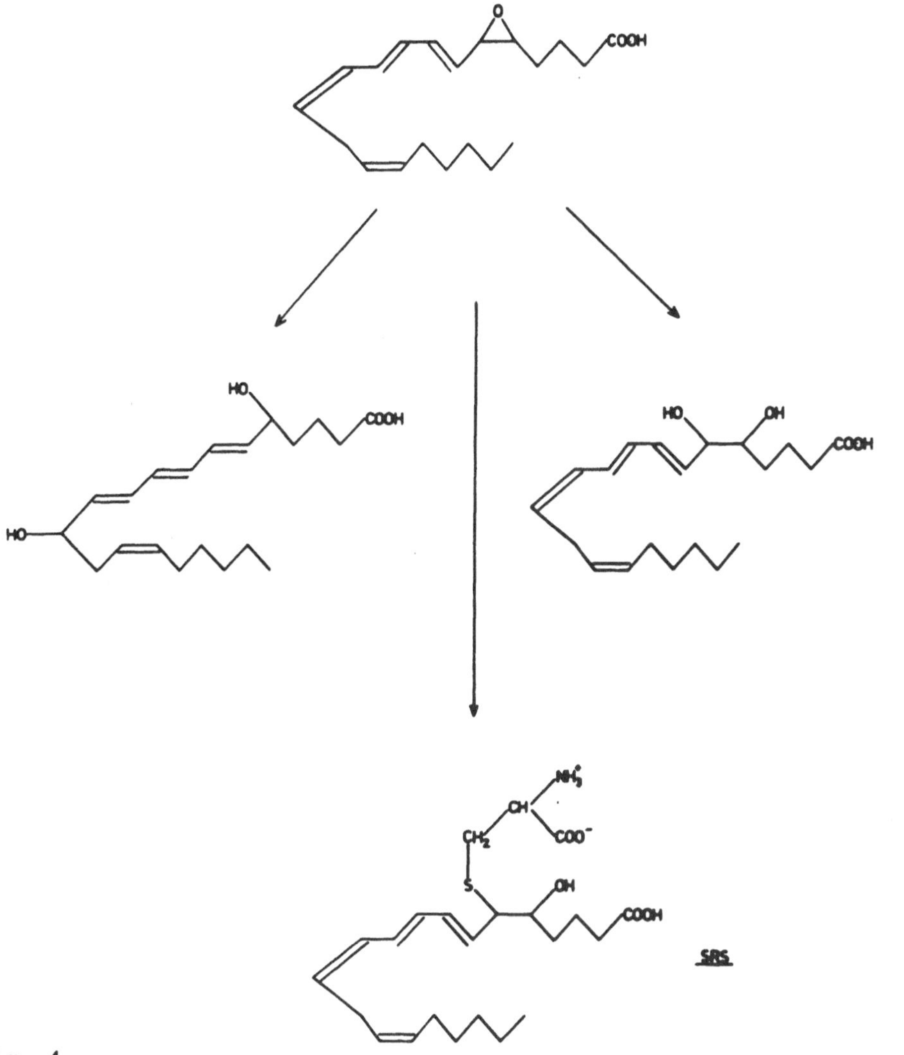

Fig. 4

The conjugated triene epoxide (upper formula) is derived from arachidonic acid via a 5-hydroperoxide. Addition of cysteine yields a Slow-Reacting Substance.

Action of fatty acid cyclo-oxygenase.

an unstable conjugated triene epoxide, 5,6-epoxy-eicosa-7,9,11,
14-tetraenoic acid.   Hydration gives two dihydroxy derivatives,
but a more important reaction is the addition of cysteine to the
epoxide group.   The isolated product has properties similar to
SRS-A, a highly active bronchoconstrictor which is released in
lung tissue following antigen-antibody interaction (19).   It is
to be anticipated that this exciting result will trigger off a
search for similar cysteine adducts to other arachidonate
epoxides.

        The prostaglandin endoperoxide, PGG_2, is the first
product which can be isolated from the interaction of arachidonic
acid and 'prostaglandin synthetase' (20).   The primary attack is
thought to occur at C11 (Fig.5) (5,6).   The next steps involve
attack of the 11-peroxy radical at C9, cyclization, shift of the
14,15 double bond and hydroperoxidation at C15 to produce the
cyclic endoperoxide PGG_2.   The 15-hydroperoxy group can be
readily reduced to a 15-hydroxyl giving PGH_2 (20,21).   The
cyclic endoperoxides are important intermediates since they can
be transformed enzymatically into several other prostaglandin
types with distinctive biological actions (22,23,24).

REFERENCES

(1)   THEORELL,H., HOLMAN,R.T. and ÅKESON,Å. (1947)   Arch.
           Biochem., 14, 250-252.

(2)   CHRISTOPHER,J.P., PISTORIUS,E.K. and AXELROD,B. (1970)
           Biochim.Biophys.Acta, 198, 12-19.

(3)   CHRISTOPHER,J.P., PISTORIUS,E.K., REGNIER,F.E. and
           AXELROD,B. (1972) Biochim.Biophys.Acta, 289, 82-87.

(4)   HAMBERG,M. and SAMUELSSON,B. (1967a).   J.Biol.Chem.,
           242, 5329-5335.

(5)   HAMBERG,M. and SAMUELSSON,B. (1967b)   J.Biol.Chem.,
           242, 5336-5343.

(6)   HAMBERG,M. and SAMUELSSON,B. (1967c)   J.Biol.Chem.,
           242, 5344-5354.

(7)   BILD,G.S., RAMADOSS,C.S. and AXELROD,B. (1977)   Arch.
           Biochem.Biophys., 184, 36-41.

(8)   BILD,G.S., BHAT,S.G., RAMADOSS,C.S., AXELROD,B. and
           SWEELEY,C.C. (1978) Biochem.Biophys.Res.Commun., 81,
           486-492.

(9)   PACE-ASCIAK,C. (1971)   Biochemistry, 10, 3664-3669.

(10)   HAMBERG,M. and SAMUELSSON,B. (1974)   Proc.Nat.Acad.Sci.

         U.S.A., 71, 3400-3404.

(11)   NUGTEREN,D.H. (1975) Biochim.Biophys.Acta, 280,
         299-307.

(12)   HAMBERG,M. (1975) Lipids, 10, 87-92.

(13)   GARDNER,H.W. (1975) J.Agr.Food Chem., 23, 129-136.

(14)   WALKER,I.C., JONES,R.L., KERRY,P.J. and WILSON,N.H.
         (1979) Prostaglandins, in press.

(15)   TURNER,S.R., TAINER,J.A. and LYNN,W.S. (1975) Nature,
         257, 680-681.

(16)   JONES,R.L., KERRY,P.J., PYSER,N.L., WALKER,I.C. and
         WILSON,N.H. (1978) Prostaglandins, 16, 583-588.

(17)   JONES,R.L., KERRY,P.J., PYSER,N.L., WALKER,I.C. and
         WILSON,N.H. (1979). In "Chemistry, Biochemistry and
         Pharmacological Activity of Prostanoids".   Ed.
         Roberts,S.M. and Scheinmann,F., pp.139-149.   Pergamon
         Press, Oxford.

(18)   SAMUELSSON,B. (1979) Proceedings of Fourth Inter-
         national Prostaglandin Conference.   Washington,D.C.,
         May 27-31, 1979.   To be published.

(19)   KELLAWAY,C.H. and THETHEWIE   (1940) Quart.J.Exptl.
         Physiol., 30, 121-145.

(20)   HAMBERG,M., SVENSSON,J., WAKABAYASHI,T. and SAMUEL-
         SSON,B. (1974) Proc.Nat.Acad.Sci., U.S.A., 71,
         345-349.

(21)   NUGTEREN,D.H. and HAZELHOF,E. (1973) Biochim.Biophys.
         Acta, 326, 448-461.

(22)   SAMUELSSON,B. (1977) In"Prostaglandin Research".
         Ed.Crabbé,P. Vol.36,pp.17-46.   Academic Press, New
         York.

(23)   DORP,D.A. van (1979) In "Chemistry, Biochemistry and
         Pharmacological Activity of Prostanoids".   Ed.Roberts,
         S.M. and Scheinmann,F., pp.233-243.   Pergamon Press,
         Oxford.

(24)   MONCADA,S. and VANE,J.R. (1979) In "Chemistry, Bio-
         chemistry and Pharmacological Activity of Prostanoids".
         Ed. Roberts,S.M. and Scheinmann,F., pp.258-273.
         Pergamon Press, Oxford.

SLOW-REACTING SUBSTANCE OF ANAPHYLAXIS: STUDIES ON
PURIFICATION AND CHARACTERISATION.

H.R. Morris, G.W. Taylor, Priscilla J. Piper and J.R. Tippins
Department of Biochemistry,
Imperial College of Science and Technology.
Department of Pharmacology,
Royal College of Surgeons of England.

Slow-reacting substance of anaphylaxis (SRS-A) is a
primary mediator of immediate-type hypersensitivity reactions,
probably playing a major role in allergic bronchospasm in man.
The biological properties and criteria for identification of SRS-A used in our studies are given in Table 1.
We have been active in the purification and structure
elucidation of SRS-A (and non-immunologically produced slow-
reacting substances - SRS's) and report here further studies
on the genesis, purification and structural properties of
guinea-pig SRS-A.

TABLE 1

Biological properties of SRS-A

1. Contracts   (i) guinea-pig ileum - longitudinal smooth
                     muscle
                (ii) guinea-pig trachea
               (iii) human bronchus
2. Releases prostaglandins and thromboxanes from guinea-pig
    lung.
3. Antagonised by FPL 55712
4. Destroyed by arylsulphatase
5. Destroyed by plant and mammalian lipoxygenases

RELEASE OF SRS-A

        The immunological release of SRS-A is affected by
drugs which modify the mobilisation or metabolism of
arachidonic acid.   Indomethacin blocks metabolism of arachidonic acid to prostaglandins by inhibiting cyclo-oxygenase
and has been shown to increase SRS-A release (1), whereas
5,8,11,14 eicosatetraynoic acid (ETA), an irreversible
inhibitor of both cyclo-oxygenase and lipoxygenase (2),
markedly reduces SRS-A output; arachidonic acid itself
potentiates SRS-A release.   It appears that SRS-A is a
product of the action of a lipoxygenase-like enzyme on
arachidonic acid, and we present further evidence for this
below.
        The effect of a series of unsaturated fatty acids on
SRS-A release from chopped lung has been investigated;   we
have shown that only those acids which may act as substrates
for platelet arachidonate lipoxygenase (3) cause potentiation
of SRS-A release (4) and that maximum potentiation occurs with

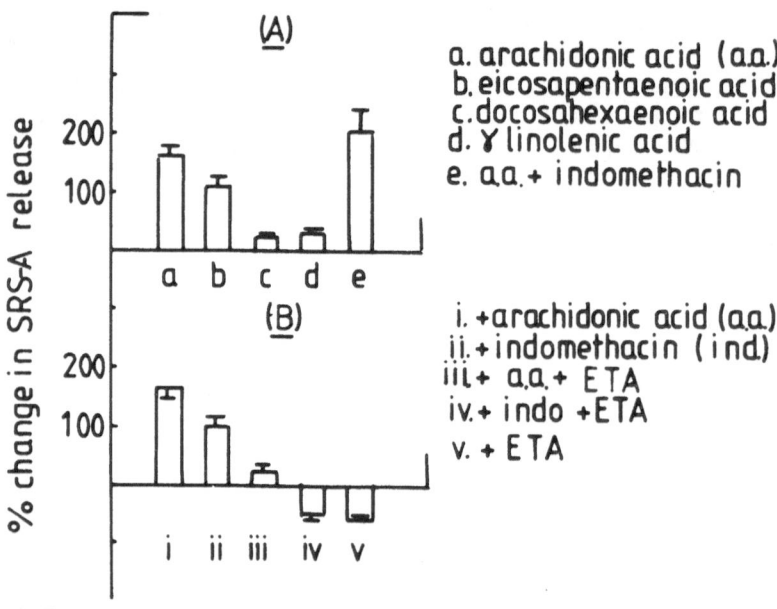

Fig. 1.

(A) The effect of fatty acids on the release of SRS-A
(B) The effect of lipoxygenase and cyclo-oxygenase-inhibiting
    drugs on the release of SRS-A

arachidonic and 5,8,11,14,17 eicosapentaenoic acids (Fig.1).
This potentiation is enhanced by indomethacin and completely
reversed by ETA as would be expected if lipoxygenase were
involved in SRS-A release.

We have not, however, been able to incorporate ^{14}C-
arachidonic acid into SRS-A (as may have been expected from
the above potentiation data); this is in agreement with other
work (5) showing that ^{14}C-arachidonic acid may be incorporated
into phospholipids, but is not mobilised on antigen challenge.
Our inability to incorporate labelled material into SRS-A is
not incompatible with our proposal that the C_{20} chain is the
skeleton of the SRS-A structure, as potentiation of SRS-A
release may be through displacement of endogenous fatty acid
at the site of action, thus precluding incorporation of
exogenous label.   It is possible that, based on a specific
activity of SRS-A much greater than previously expected, (e.g.
a minimum level of detection of 10 pg or less), that ^{14}C
incorporation, if present, would not be observed.

Further evidence for the class of compound is the
destruction of biological activity by both plant (6) and
mammalian (7) lipoxygenases of varying positional specificity;
these enzymes attack arachidonic-related compounds containing
cis-1-4-diene systems suggesting the probably presence of such
a unit in SRS-A.

CHEMICAL PROPERTIES

The chemical properties of SRS-A are outlined in
Table 2 and are consistent with an unsaturated lipid containing
hydroxyl, carboxyl and amino groups (short acetylation data)
and thioether linkages.   The presence of a sulphate moeity
in the molecule (8) is brought into question by the solubility
of SRS-A in ether at pH 3; it would be expected that such a
group would remain unprotonated at this pH and thus remain in
the aqueous phase.   The possibility, however, of ion pairing
with, for example, an amino group removing the effect of a
negative charge (thus enhancing ether solubility), cannot be
discounted.

TABLE 2

Chemical properties of SRS-A

1.   Biological activity is stable to:
        (i) boiling
        (ii) base treatment, 0.1 M NaOH, RT, 30 mins
     (iii) sodium borohydride reduction.
2.   Biological activity is destroyed by:
        (i) HCl, 0.1 M, RT, 30 mins.
        (ii) Acetylation: MeOH-Acetic anydride 4/1 v/v 1 min.
      (iii) fluram treatment
       (iv) Methylation: $CH_2 N_2$, RT, 30 mins.
                         MeOH/HCl, RT, 30 mins.
                         MeOH/BF_3, 37°C, 30 mins.
        (v) Catalytic hydrogenation, $N_2 B$, RT and 55°C, 30 mins.
            in MeOH
       (vi) CNBr treatment
3.   Water soluble at pH 7
     Ether soluble at pH 3
     Migrates anodically on HVPE at pH 6.5

PURIFICATION

        We have developed a rapid purification procedure
for SRS-A (and related SRS's) involving reverse-phase high-
pressure liquid chromatography (HPLC) leading to completely
pure SRS-A, and related compounds, in ug quantities.   We
have recently extended our original purification (9) to
include a further reverse-phase HPLC step using n-propanol:
acetic acid:water as eluant (5,11).   HPLC elution profiles
are given in Fig.2.

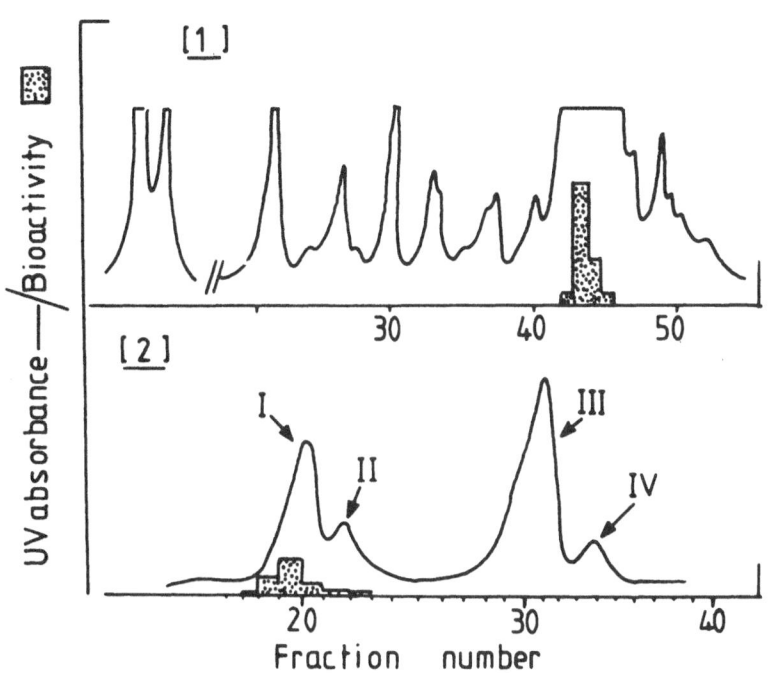

Fig.2.   HPLC profile of guinea-pig SRS-A (μ Bondapak C$_{18}$
          column)
          1. methanol:water gradient. 50% methanol:water,
              5 mins isocratically followed by a 10 min linear
              gradient to 100% methanol
          2. n-propanol:acetic acid:water gradient. 30% n-
              propanol in 5% aqueous acetic acid,10 mins iso-
              cratically followed by a 20 min linear gradient
              to 40% n-propanol in acetic acid

          In the second HPLC step (HPLC 2) biological activity
co-elutes with u.v. absorbance (280nm) and is well separated
from other u.v. absorbing materials.   The full u.v. spectrum
of the biologically active material (I) (published previously
(9)) shows a broad triplet λ_{max}^{MeOH} 280 ± 1nm with shoulders at
270 and 290 nm (Fig.3); the spectrum is not affected by

addition of mild acid or base.   Comparison of our spectrum
with that published by Bild et al (11) for lipoxygenase-
derived arachidonic acid metabolites led us to the conclusion
that SRS-A contains a conjugated triene system.
        Eluting immediately after SRS-A in HPLC 2 is a
weakly biologically-active material (II) whose u.v. spectrum
resembles that of SRS-A but is shifted hypsochromically by
3nm (Fig. 3); this would be in accordance with a cis/trans
isomerisation or other very closely related structural
change.   Such modification could be expected to reduce
biological activity as is observed.   The identification of
this material is at present under study.

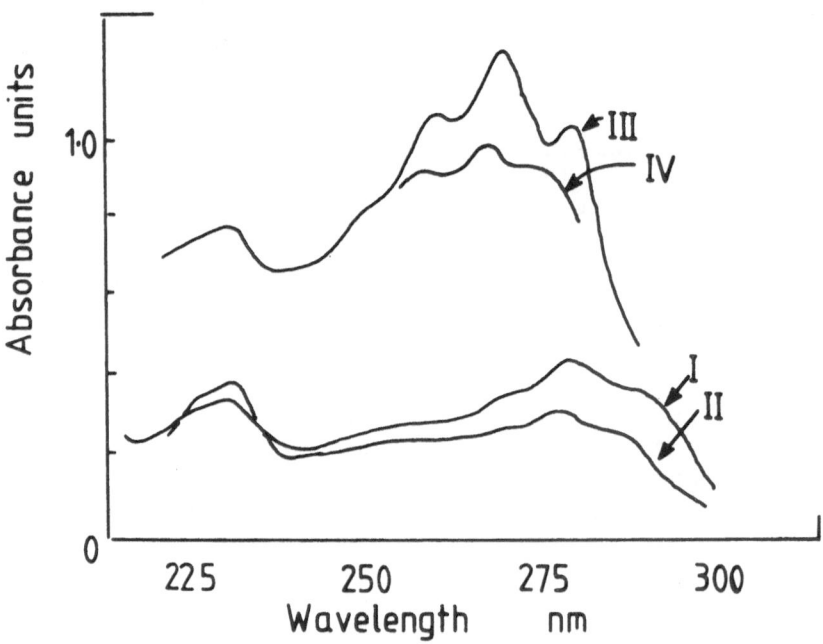

Fig. 3.   Full ultra-violet spectrum of ex HPLC 2 samples in
          methanol.

        Two compounds (III,IV) again related to each other
by a 3nm shift in the u.v. elute somewhat later than SRS-A,
but have no biological activity; the first compound has a
full u.v. spectrum consistent with a cis trans trans or
similar triene (λ max 270 nm), with the latter compound
possibly corresponding to the all trans triene (12).   Mass
spectrometric evidence (of the trimethylsilyl derivative
of the carboxylic methyl ester) is interpreted as originating
from 5,12 dihydroxy-eicosatetraenoic acid (Fig. 4).   This is
the first report of this novel arachidonic acid metabolite
being liberated from lung on antigen challenge.   The mass
spectrum of the related compound referred to above shows a
different fragmentation pattern and is presently under
investigation.

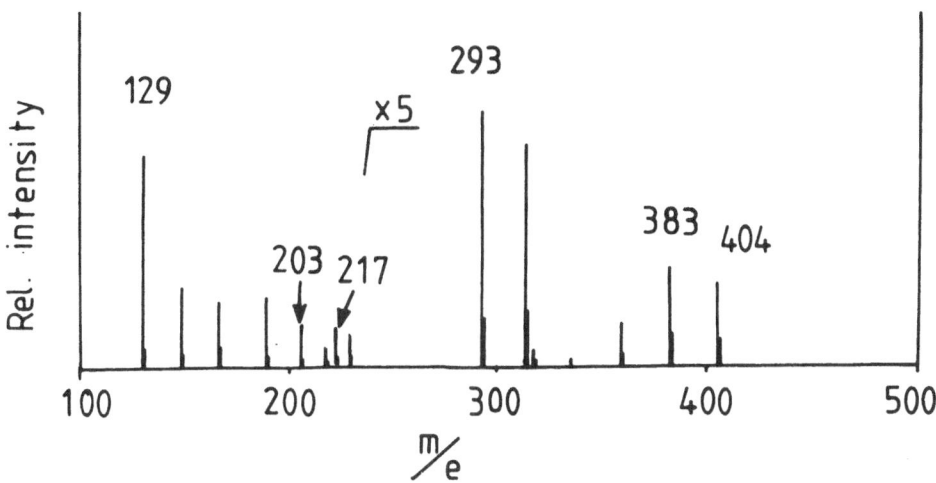

Fig.4.   E.I. mass spectrum of the trimethylsilyl derivative
         of the methyl ester of compound III (ex HPLC 2).
         High temperature silylation in pyridine:BSTFA:TMCS.
         Source temperature 200 C.
         No molecular ion was observed due to facile elimina-
         tion of TMS-OH under the derivative-forming
         conditions used.

Recently an SRS has been released from murine mastocytoma cells and its structure has been reported as 5-hydroxy-6-L-cysteinyl-7,8,11,14-eicosatetraenoic acid (13) (Fig. 5).   This material has a u.v. absorbance spectrum similar to that reported for SRS-A (9).

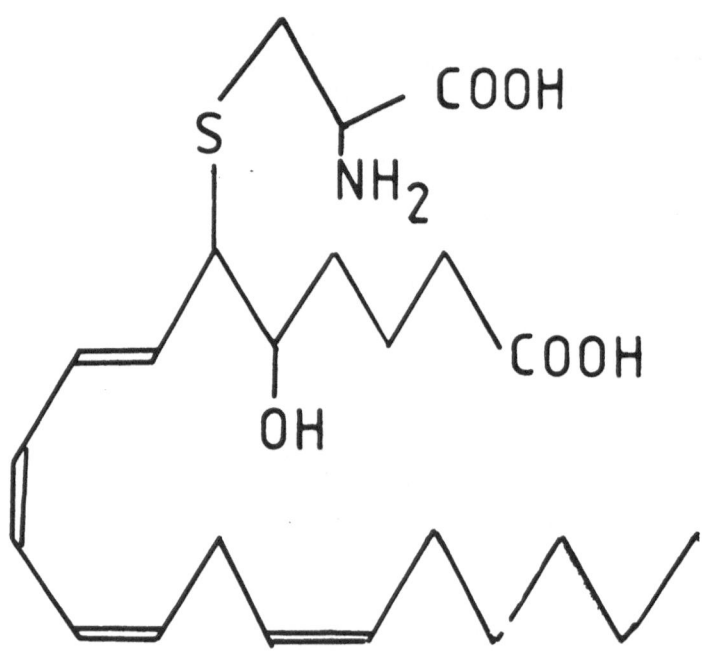

Fig. 5.   Structure of Leucotriene C from Samuelsson 1979 (13)

Our own structural data on SRS-A may be summarised as follows: we have strong biological evidence for the involvement of arachidonic acid, and chemical / spectroscopic evidence for the conjugated triene and cis 1,4 diene in the structure.   Chemical de-activation experiments indicate the possible presence of an α-amino group and a thioether linkage. We have identified the mass spectrum of a material closely related to SRS-A by its u.v. spectrum and HPLC profile (III) as 5,12 di-hydroxy-6,8,10,14 eicosatetraenoic acid.   Our

independent evidence is therefore consistent with the structure shown in Fig. 5, however, the mass spectrum of a
derivative of our active material cannot at present be
interpreted as arising from this structure. A full interpre-
tation of our data is still in progress and is constrained by
the very low levels of material (we estimate ug quantities)
purified from several hundred animals.
        We have shown (14) that both immunologically (in
particular human material) and non-immunologically released
forms of SRS-A are pharmacologically, chemically and chromato-
graphically identical, we are now confirming these studies on
our newly developed HPLC purification procedure.

CONCLUSION

        We have demonstrated the role of arachidonic acid
and lipoxygenase in the genesis of SRS-A and the possible
role of lipoxygenases in its metabolism.   SRS-A has been
purified in μg quantities together with closely related
material.   We have identified 5,12 di-hydroxy-6,8,10,14
eicosatetraenoic acid released by antigen challenge, and
which we feel is related to SRS-A.   Further structural
work is in progress.

REFERENCES

1. Engineer, D.M., Niederhauser, U., Piper, P.J. & Sirois,P.
    (1978) Br.J.Pharmac., 62, 61-66.
2. Jakschik, B.A., Falkenhein, S. and Parker, C.W. (1977)
    Proc.Natl.Acad.Sci. (USA), 74, 4577-4581.
3. Nugteren, D.H. (1975) Biochem.biophys.Acta, 380,299-307.
4. Piper, P.J., Morris, H.R., Tippins, J.R. & Taylor, G.W.
    (1979) Advances in Prostaglandins and Thromboxanes
    Research (in press)
5. Jose, P.J. & Seale, J.P. (1979) Br.J.Pharmac., (in press)
6. Engineer, D.M., Morris, H.R., Piper, P.J. & Sirois, P.
    (1978) Br.J.Pharmac., 64, 211-218.
7. Piper, P.J. & Tippins, J.R. (unpublished results)
8. Orange, R.P., Murphy, R.C. & Austen, K.F. (1974) J.Immunol.
    113, 316-322.

9.   Morris, H.R., Taylor, G.W., Piper, P.J., Sirois, P.
      & Tippins, J.R. (1978) FEBS Letters, 87, 203-206.
10.   Piper, P.J., Tippins, J.R., Morris, H.R. & Taylor, G.W.
      (1979) Prostaglandins (in press)
11.   Bild, G.S., Ramadoss, C.S., Lim, S. & Axelrod, B. (1977)
      Biochem. biophys. res.commun., 74, 949-954.
12.   Morton, R.A. in: Comprehensive Biochemistry, ed. Florkin
      M. & Stotz, E. Chapter IV, pp 99-105.
13.   Samuelsson, B. (1979) Advances in Prostaglandins and
      Thromboxane Research (in press)
14.   Morris. H.R., Piper, P.J., Taylor, G.W. & Tippins, J.R.
      (1979) Br.J.Pharmac., (in press)

Slow-reacting substances of anaphylaxis - a commentary.
W. Brokelhurst, Scripps Institute, La Jolla, California, USA.

The statement that the pharmacology reported by various workers refers
to SRS-A which has been only partially purified is obviously true, but the
reliability of the data may be much better than has been inferred. It hap-
pens that the pharmacological effects of SRS-A are very few and remarkably
selective. Outstanding selective effects of SRS-A are evident in the guinea-
pig ileum and human bronchial muscle. In other tissues, e.g. the guinea-pig
airways muscle and the rat gastric muscle the effect(s) may be indirect. All
other tissues tested have failed to respond until the dose was raised to
such a level where effects of impurities could induce artefacts. The tissues
which do not respond to SRS-A include all preparations of uterus and vascular
tissue and most gut preparations. This lack of activity was originally used
to justify the conclusion that SRS-A was different from other "known"
substances (including those having the generic description "SRS"). Also, it
shows that the samples of SRS-A used must have been free from the long list
of autocoids known to act on these tissues.

Recognising the lack of methods to remove possible artefactual contaminants, most of the early studies used only samples collected at strategic
times from perfused lung. This avoided much of the antigen in early samples
and products of tissue damage in "late" fractions. Qualitative pharmacological data from such material has never been called in question. However,
the quantitative data is less reliable because enhancement of the bioassay
occurs with contaminants such as histamine, kinins and prostaglandins. Also,
the activity of SRS-A preparations is reduced in the presence of proteins
and lipids. It follows that any biological comparison of SRS-A from different sources (each with different contaminants), is difficult. Moreover,
the narrow spectrum of biological activity has handicapped parallel quantitative assays which are the usual standby.

Fortunately, the very selective biological properties of SRS-A should
be a blessing to those who wish to compare SRS-A preparations with a
synthetic product, or to relate physical measurements to biological activity.
I think that at this important stage in the story of SRS-A it is imperative
that a wide range of biological tests be used to support any statement
concerning the chemistry of SRS-A. These tests should show the specificity
of biological activity currently recognised for SRS-A as well as selective
inhibition and destruction of the activity.

I am concerned that physico-chemical data obtained by Dr. Morris, and
others, does not agree with that obtained by Dr. Dawson. For instance,
Dr. Dawson has not observed a conjugated double bond system in SRS-A as
indicated by NMR & UV spectroscopy. I believe that the preparation used by
Dr. Dawson's group was 10,000 units/μg, suggesting that this material has
apparently high specific activity.

PEROXIDASE REACTIONS DURING PROSTAGLANDIN BIOSYNTHESIS
AND THEIR RELATIONSHIP TO INFLAMMATION

by

Robert W. Egan, Paul H. Gale, William J. A. VandenHeuvel
and Frederick A. Kuehl, Jr.

Merck Institute for Therapeutic Research
Rahway, New Jersey 07065

Peroxidase activity plays a significant role in
prostaglandin biosynthesis, catalyzing the reduction of PGG_2
to either PGH_2 or 15-hydroperoxyPGE$_2$ (1-5). Positioned as
it is in the arachidonic acid cascade, this enzyme may
regulate the absolute and relative quantities of prostaglandins and thromboxanes formed. Both peroxidase and fatty
acid oxygenase activities appear to be associated with a
single protein called either prostaglandin cyclooxygenase or
endoperoxide synthetase (6,7). This bifunctional enzyme has
been purified and shown to possess heme groups (8-10) which
are probably involved with its catalytic activity. This
manuscript describes both some recently discovered aspects of
peroxidase reactions and a relationship between peroxidases,
radical scavenging and depression of inflammation.

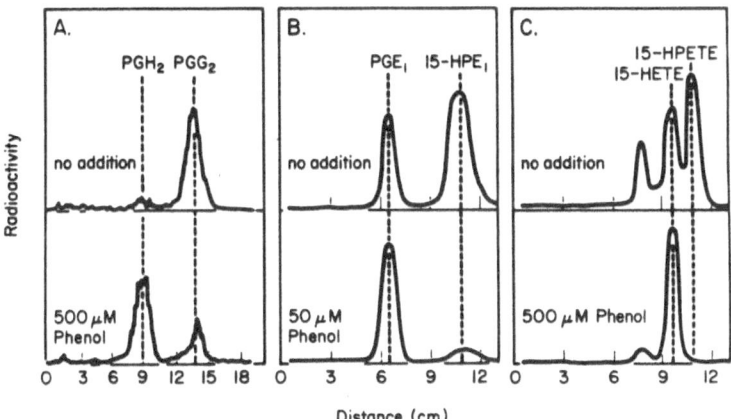

Figure 1. Metabolism of [^{14}C]Hydroperoxides by Vesicular
Gland Peroxidase. A) Reaction at 25° for 30 sec with 24 µM
PGG$_2$ and 0.05 mg microsomal protein. Chromatography with
ether/hexane/acetic acid (85:15:0.1). B) Reaction at 25° for
60 sec with 71 µM 15-HPE$_1$ and 0.5 mg microsomal protein.
Chromatography with ether/methanol/acetic acid (90:1:2).
C) Reaction at 25° for 60 sec with 112 µM 15-HPETE and
0.5 mg microsomal protein. Chromatography with isopropyl
ether/methyl ethyl ketone/acetic acid (50:50:1).

    The selectivity of this peroxidase for hydroperoxide
substrate is rather broad, with PGG$_2$, 15-hydroperoxyPGE1
(15-HPE$_1$) and 15-hydroperoxyeicosatetraenoic acid (15-HPETE)
serving this function (Fig. 1). These are radiochromatograms
of the reaction products when [^{14}C]hydroperoxide was incubated
with ram seminal vesicle microsomes, followed by acidification
and solvent extraction (4). Phenol enhanced each of these
reactions (lower panels), promoting the conversions of PGG$_2$
to PGH$_2$, 15-HPE$_1$ to PGE$_1$ and 15-HPETE to 15-hydroxyeicosa-
tetraenoic acid (15-HETE). Even H$_2$O$_2$ will be reduced by this
enzyme, although its preference for hydrophobic peroxides is
perhaps a reflection of its membraneous environment.

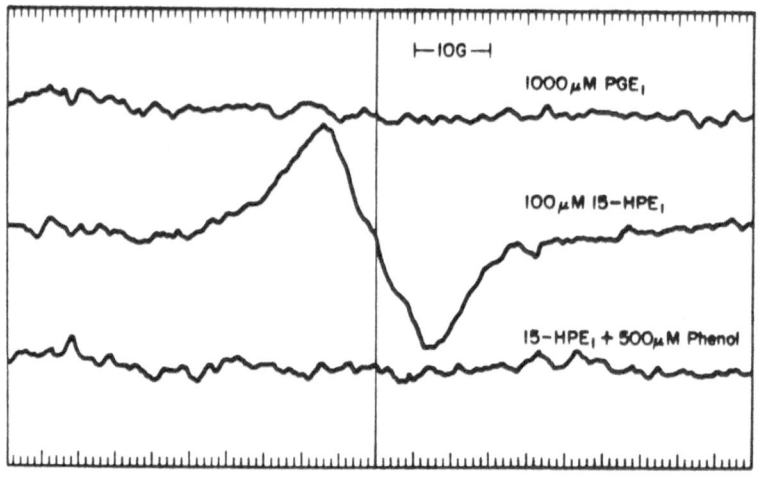

Figure 2. Peroxidase-catalyzed Electron Spin Resonance
Signal from 15-HPE$_1$. Reaction with 4 mg microsomal protein
for 30 sec at 25°. Sample frozen at -196° and scanned at
-185° over a 200 G scan range centered at g=2.

The radical generated enzymatically with arachidonic acid and PGG_2 (2), was also observed with each hydroperoxide substrate and the resulting EPR signal is shown in Fig. 2 for enzyme and $15-HPE_1$. Signals were obtained when the reaction was frozen at the peak of activity and the sample was analyzed in the spectrometer at $-185°C$. This broad, rather non-descript peak was depressed by phenol and other radical-scavenging reducing agents and was the same for each hydroperoxide. Furthermore, it has been demonstrated that the oxidant responsible for generating it can lead to irreversible in-activation of the cyclooxygenase (2), the peroxidase (4), PGI_2 synthetase (11) and perhaps to generalized cellular damage. Hence, we interpret the apparent stimulatory aspects of radical-scavenging reducing agents in terms of their capacity to be oxidized in place of and thereby preserve the enzymes, leading to increased reaction.

Table 1

Stimulation of Hydroperoxide Metabolism by Cosubstrates

Cosubstrate	Cosubstrate Concentration	Percentage Change [a]		
		PGG_2	$15-HPE_1$	15-HPETE
	(µM)			
Phenol	500	+610	+275	+290
Aminopyrine	1000	+570	+307	+150
Diethyldithiocarbamate	200	+480	+274	+188
Promethazine	100	+525	+264	+179
Sulindac sulfide	100	+525	+257	+178
Lipoic acid	100	+465	+228	+306
Methional	200	+345	+111	+39
Tryptophan	500	+130	+57	+100
Anisole	2000	-10	-5	-27
Salicylic acid	2000	+10	-5	+9
Glutathione (red)	500	-	-5	-18
Methionine	500	-20	-7	0
Sulindac	2000	+10	-8	+6
Indomethacin	500	0	-31	-17

[a] plus indicates stimulation and minus indicates inhibition of the reaction relative to control incubations containing no cosubstrate.

To help clarify whether the same enzyme was involved
in each reaction, the cosubstrate dependence was established
for all three hydroperoxides as shown in Table 1.   The extent
of reaction was measured using the incubation procedure
described above and percentage change was determined relative
to a control with no additive.   It can be seen by comparing
the columns of percentage change for the three hydroperoxides
that each cosubstrate influenced all three reactions in an
identical manner.   Those compounds above the dotted line,
phenol, aminopyrine, diethyldithiocarbamate, promethazine,
sulindac sulfide, lipoic acid, methional and tryptophan,
stimulated in each instance while those below the line,
anisole, salicylic acid, reduced glutathione, methionine,
sulindac and indomethacin had either no significant effect
or mild inhibition.   Based on this evidence, the same enzyme
is certainly reducing each hydroperoxide.

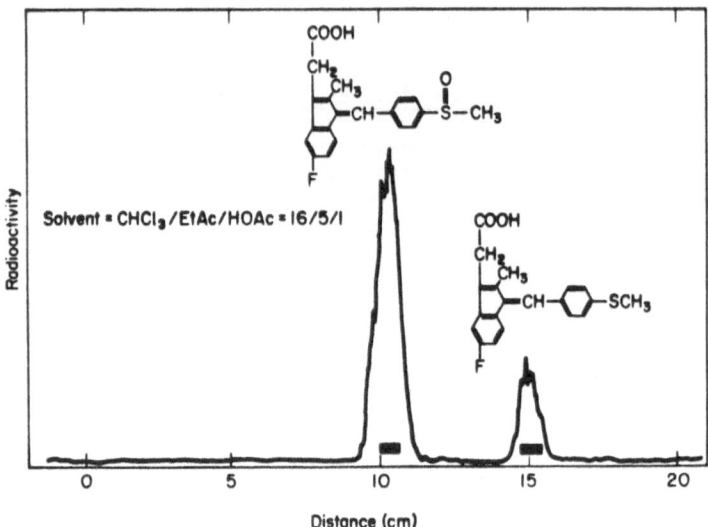

Figure 3.   Radiochromatogram of Peroxidase-catalyzed
Sulindac Sulfide Metabolism.   Reaction at 25° for 60 sec
with 100 μM [3H]sulindac sulfide, 150 μM 15-HPE$_1$ and 0.56 mg
microsomal protein.   Bars at 10 and 15 cm indicate standards.
Structures are above the appropriate peaks, sulindac at 10 cm
and sulindac sulfide at 15 cm.

    To examine the role of reducing cosubstrate in detail,
we will focus on two of these compounds, sulindac sulfide
which was active and sulindac which was not. In its capacity
as cosubstrate for the peroxidase, sulindac sulfide, itself,
should be oxidized and Fig. 3 shows the metabolism of [^{3}H]-
sulindac sulfide during peroxidatic reduction of 15-HPE$_1$ to
PGE$_1$. This figure is a radiochromatogram of the reaction
products with the structures above the peaks which indicate
the amount of that material in the mixture. The sulfide was
converted exclusively to the inactive sulfoxide with an
optimal stoichiometry of one-to-one between 15-HPE$_1$ and
sulfide. The reaction was protein dependent, destroyed by
heat denaturation and elicited by PGG$_2$, 15-HPETE and H$_2$O$_2$ as
well as 15-HPE$_1$. Furthermore, there was competition between
sulindac sulfide and microsomal tissue for the oxidant (4),
in keeping with the postulate that enzymes can be attacked
by nascent oxidizing species generated by the peroxidase (2).

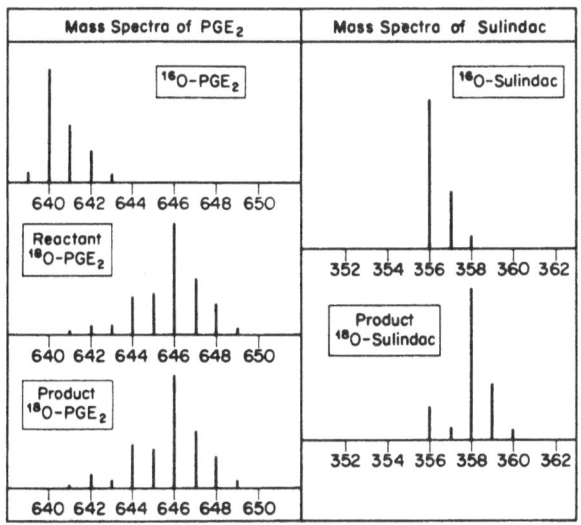

Figure 4. Mass Spectra of ^{18}O-Labeled Peroxidase Reaction
Products. Peroxidase reaction used 250 µM [^{18}O]15-HPE$_2$,
150 µM sulindac sulfide and 4 mg microsomal protein in 1 ml
of potassium phosphate buffered at pH 7.0. Incubation was
for 60 sec at 25°. Mass spectra were obtained using the
direct inlet system on a LKB 7000 mass spectrometer with tri-
methylsilylated PGE$_2$ and untreated sulindac sulfide.

The actual mechanism of oxygen transfer to the sulfide
has been examined by mass spectral determination of the
distribution of oxygen-18 in the products, with $[^{18}O]$15-HPE$_2$
as reactant (12). Labeled 15-HPE$_2$ was prepared by the cyclooxygenase-catalyzed reaction of arachidonic acid with $^{18}O_2$
in the presence of 1 mM reduced glutathione. An 18% yield
of 15-HPE$_2$ was obtained along with about 16% PGE$_2$. Because
of the dioxygenase reaction mechanism, the isotopic composition
of the 15-HPE$_2$ and PGE$_2$ would be identical and the PGE$_2$ was
used to establish this parameter because it produced a more
interpretable mass spectrum (Fig. 4). Mass spectra for the
tetra-trimethylsilylated derivatives of both enzymatically-
prepared (middle panel) and authentic (upper panel) PGE$_2$
were the basis for comparison. The molecular ion for
authentic PGE$_2$ was 640, the largest peak in this region.
Since the labeled PGE$_2$ could contain either zero, one, two
or three ^{18}O-atoms, the ratios of 640, 642, 644 and 646 were
compared to establish the isotopic distribution which showed
that 78% of the hydroxyl at carbon-15 contained ^{18}O-atoms.
The presence of ^{16}O-atoms in this sample reflects the inadvertent
presence of $^{16}O_2$ in the starting gas. Consequently, 78% of
the 15-HPE$_2$ would possess ^{18}O-atoms in the hydroperoxide.

Labeled 15-HPE$_2$ was then used as hydroperoxide substrate
for the cyclooxygenase-catalyzed oxidation of sulindac sulfide
to sulindac. Following one minute of reaction at room
temperature, the products and remaining substrates were
acidified, extracted into ether, backwashed with water and
separated by TLC. The PGE$_2$ resulting from this reaction
(lower panel) showed 75% oxygen-18 at carbon 15 compared with
78% in the starting 15-HPE$_2$. This excellent agreement confirms
that the hydroperoxide moiety was not exchanging in some
unexpected fashion.

The sulindac formed was also subjected to mass spectral
analysis to determine the percentage of oxygen-18 in the
sulfoxide, as shown on the right hand panels of Fig. 4.
Since authentic sulindac (upper panel) had a large 356 peak
(the molecular ion), a small 358 peak and no 354 peak, $[^{18}O]$-
sulindac would have a large 358 peak and no 356 peak. By
comparing the intensities at 356 and 358, an isotopic
distribution of 78% $[^{18}O]$ and 22% $[^{16}O]$ was established for
the sulfoxide in the enzymatically prepared sulindac (lower
panel). Since this was identical to the distribution in the
15-HPE$_2$ reactant, each oxygen atom transferred to the sulfide
originated exclusively with the hydroperoxide.

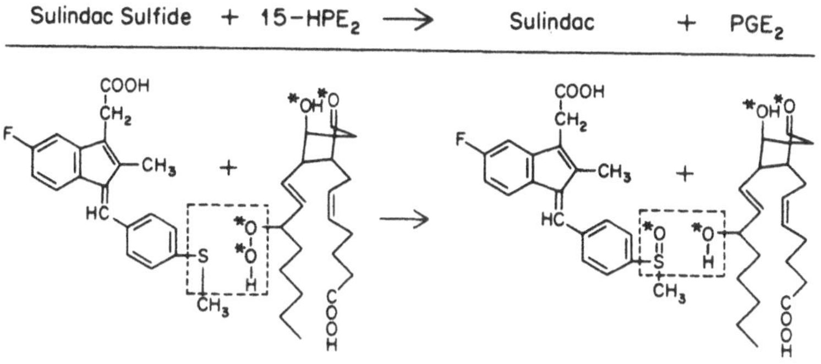

Figure 5.   Mechanism of Sulindac Sulfide Oxidation.

    This reaction is depicted in detail in Fig. 5.   There
was a stoichiometric equimolar reaction between sulindac
sulfide and 15-HPE$_2$, a stoichiometry which could be altered
by introducing other oxidizable agents to compete with
sulindac sulfide.   The structures are shown below the
equation with the functional groups placed in proximity,
enclosed within a dashed box and asterisks designating
oxygen-18 atoms.   The oxygen atom was transferred to the
sulfide and, following the reaction, all the atoms were
accounted for precluding indirect oxidizing species such
as molecular or singlet oxygen as contributors to this
cooxygenation.   This is not true of all substrates since
Marnett (5) has shown that diphenylisobenzofuran was
oxygenated by this same enzyme in a chain reaction using
dissolved molecular oxygen.   Whether the intermediate in
this transfer is enzyme-bound as in a typical peroxidase
ferryl or perferryl ion or is free as a radical in
solution has not yet been established.

<u>Catalase</u>

$$H_2O_2 \longrightarrow O_2 + H_2O$$

<u>Glutathione Peroxidase</u>

$$ROOH + GSH \longrightarrow ROH + GSSG$$

<u>Multisubstrate Oxidizing Peroxidases</u>
(MOPS)

$$ROOH \longrightarrow ROH + [O_x] \xrightarrow{AH} A + [O_x]H$$

<u>Figure 6</u>. Classification of Peroxidases. GSH and GSSG
are reduced and oxidized by glutathione respectively. R
is an alkyl group or hydrogen and AH is an oxidizable
molecule with an oxidized form, A.

A characteristic of the class of peroxidases we are
investigating is shown in Fig. 6, a class which I have
termed multisubstrate oxidizing peroxidases and abbreviated
MOPS. Whereas the function of catalase is to dispose of
hydrogen peroxide to less potentially toxic materials and
glutathione peroxidase also does this using reduced glutathione as specific reducing cosubstrate, the MOPS enzymes
cleave the peroxide bond in such a way that highly reactive
and potentially toxic oxidizing species, $[O_x]$, are generated.
These could react with any of a variety of cellular
constituents in non-constructive fashion. Therefore, rather
than removing potentially toxic peroxides, MOPS enzymes, of
which prostaglandin peroxidase is one, would actually form
toxic moieties in response to appropriate stimuli. Although
these reactions have been defined with lipid hydroperoxides,
H_2O_2 is also a substrate for these enzymes and could arise
from a large variety of sources within the cell.

This suggested that the oxidizing species generated
during these peroxidase reactions could be responsible for
some of the symptoms of an inflammatory lesion. If true,
then any enzyme in the MOPS classification should possess
these characteristics. Evidence in support of this concept

for the prostaglandin cyclooxygenase was published in 1977
(13) and is shown diagrammatically in Table 2.   Inflammation
was measured as the edema induced by irritating the ear of
a mouse with phorbol myristate acetate.   The other principle
symptoms of inflammation, pain and vasodilation, were not
monitored, although pain may require the same stimuli as
edema.   Vasodilation, on the other hand, is induced by PGE
alone while prostaglandins require another mediator such as
bradykinin to elicit a full edematous or algesic response (14).

Table 2

Correlation Between Antiinflammatory Activity and Prostaglandin Biosynthesis

Species	MK-447	Phenol	Anisole	Indocin	Aspirin
AA	↓ (a)	↓	−	↑	↑
PGG_2	↓	↓	−	↓	↓
PGH_2	↑	↑	−	↓	↓
PGs	↑	↑	−	↓	↓
EPR signal	↓	↓	−	↓	↓
Anti inf.	⊕	⊕	⊖	⊕	⊕

(a) Arrows represent the amount of that material in the mixture
following reaction relative to the same reaction in the
absence of any additive.

The objective was to establish a correlation between
the ability of these compounds to both dissipate edema and
to uniformly alter a parameter of prostaglandin biosynthesis.
The in vitro prostaglandin formation was monitored in ram
seminal vesicle gland microsomes.   All of these compounds
except anisole were antiedema agents and anisole did not
influence prostaglandin biosynthesis anyway.   Indomethacin
and aspirin retarded arachidionic acid utilization whereas
phenol and MK-447, 2-aminomethyl-4-t-butyl-6-iodophenol,
had the opposite effect.   Likewise, PGH_2 and PGs were
depressed by indomethacin and aspirin but augmented by the
phenols.   However, each compound depressed PGG_2 levels.   On
these grounds, we suggest that PGG_2 plays a pivotal role in

edema. The peroxidase-dependent EPR signal, an indicator
of the levels of [O_x], was also depressed by each of these
agents. This further indicated that the pivotal role of
PGG_2 was probably a function of its ability to be converted
to other substances and that during reduction of PGG_2 the
oxidizing species that was released might be an actual
inflammatory mediator.

   Under normal conditions, in vivo prostaglandin biosynthesis would be expected to proceed in a controlled
manner such that fatty acid availability would regulate
the reaction rate and any toxic group released during the
process would be detoxified by cellular constituents.
However, in a pathological state where cells are being
injured, large amounts of free fatty acid would become
available, increasing prostaglandin output and releasing
large quantities of oxidizing moieties. This could over-
whelm the cell's defenses, causing generalized cellular
damage, eventual lysis, and release of lytic enzymes such
as lysosomal components. By this method, the cellular
lysis would propagate, eventually leading to an inflamed
area. Since there are several sources of peroxide
substrate for the peroxidase, this concept may extend well
beyond prostaglandin biosynthesis, involving a series of
enzymes designated multisubstrate oxidizing peroxidases
(MOPS) which generate highly toxic species from hydroperoxides.

REFERENCES

1. Marnett, L. J., Wlodawer, P., and Samuelsson, B.
    J. Biol. Chem. 250, 8510-8517 (1975).

2. Egan, R. W., Paxton, J., and Kuehl, F. A., Jr.
    J. Biol. Chem. 251, 7329-7335 (1976).

3. O'Brien, P. J., and Rahimtula, A. Biochem. Biophys.
    Res. Commun. 70, 832-838 (1976).

4. Egan, R. W., Gale, P. H., and Kuehl, F. A., Jr.
    J. Biol. Chem. 254, 3295-3302 (1979).

5. Marnett, L. J., Bienkowski, M. J., and Pagels, W. R.
    J. Biol. Chem. 254, 5077-5082 (1979).

6. Miyamoto, T., Ogino, N., Yamamoto, S. and Hayaishi,
    O. J. Biol. Chem. 251, 2629-2636 (1976).

7. Ohki, S., Ogino, N., Yamamoto, S., and Hayaishi, O.
    J. Biol. Chem. 254, 829-836 (1979).

8. Hemler, M., Lands, W. E. M., and Smith, W. L.
    J. Biol. Chem. 251, 5575-5579 (1976).

9. Van der Ouderaa, F. J., Buytenhek, M., Nugteren,
    D. H. and Van Dorp, D. A. Biochim. Biophys. Acta
    487, 315-331 (1977).

10. Van der Ouderaa, F. J., Buytenhek, M., Slikkerveer,
    F. J. and Van Dorp, D. A. Biochim. Biophys. Acta
    572, 29-42 (1979).

11. Ham, E. A., Egan, R. W., Soderman, D. D., Gale, P. H.,
    and Kuehl, F. A., Jr. J. Biol. Chem. 254, 2191-2194
    (1979).

12. Egan, R. W., Gale, P. H., VandenHeuvel, W. J. A. and
    Kuehl, F. A., Jr. J. Biol. Chem. submitted for
    publication.

13. Kuehl, F. A., Jr., Humes, J. L., Egan, R. W., Ham,
    E. A., Beveridge, G. C. and Van Arman, C. G. Nature
    265, 170-173 (1977).

14. Ferreira, S. H., and Vane, J. R. Ann. Rev. Pharm.
    14, 57-73 (1974).

PLASMA LEVELS OF IMMUNOREACTIVE 15-KETO-13,14-DIHYDRO-THROMBOXANE B$_2$ IN GUINEA PIGS DURING ANAPHYLAXIS AND AFTER HISTAMINE INJECTION

B.A. Peskar and A. Holland

Pharmakologisches Institut der Universität Freiburg i.Br., Hermann-Herder-Str. 5, D-7800 Freiburg i.Br., F.R.G.

Summary

A sensitive radioimmunoassay for 15-keto-13,14-dihydro-thromboxane B$_2$ was developed using a monovalent iodinated tracer. The radioimmunoassay was used to determine levels of 15-keto-13, 14-dihydro-thromboxane B$_2$ in guinea pig plasma after injection of histamine and during anaphylactic shock.

Introduction

It has been shown (1) that the main product of arachidonic acid metabolism via the cyclooxygenase pathway in guinea pig lung is thromboxane A$_2$ (TXA$_2$). This compound is largely responsible for the activity of "rabbit aorta contracting substance", which is released from isolated sensitized guinea pig lungs after challenge (2). Biologically measurable amounts of TXA$_2$ are also released from guinea pig lung parenchyma by histamine (3). Since TXA$_2$ has a very short half life and is rapidly hydrolyzed to the biologically much less active TXB$_2$ (1), it seems rather difficult to measure synthesis and release of TXA$_2$ in vivo. TXB$_2$ has been determined in biological material by sensitive and specific radioimmunoassays (4-6). However, in plasma TXB$_2$ possibly represents only a minor fraction of the total TXA$_2$ released from organs, since much of the TXA$_2$ might be linked covalently to plasma proteins (7,8). Furthermore, correct plasma levels of TXB$_2$ are difficult to determine as great artifactual formation of TXB$_2$ can be expected during sampling (9). Recently Dawson et al.(10) using gas liquid chromatography/mass spectrometry have shown that large amounts of 15-keto-13,14-dihydro-TXB$_2$ (TXDK) are released from isolated perfused anaphylactic guinea pig lungs. Obviously a significant fraction of the TX synthesized after challenge is metabolized within the lung before being released into the perfusate. Similar findings have been reported previously for prostaglandin E$_2$ (PGE$_2$) and PGF$_{2\alpha}$ (11,12). We have recently described (13) a radioimmunoassay for TXDK employing a polyvalent iodinated tracer. The radioimmunoassay was

used to determine the release of TXDK from isolated organs (13).
However, the assay was not sensitive enough for in vivo studies.
We have now greatly improved the sensitivity of the radioimmunoassay for TXDK by the use of a monovalent iodinated tracer. The
improved radioimmunoassay was used for some preliminary in vivo
studies on plasma levels of TXDK in guinea pigs.

Methods

1.   Preparation of the iodinated tracer:
          The monovalent tracer for the TXDK radioimmunoassay was
prepared by a procedure similar to the one described for various
PGs and TXB_2 by Dray's group (6,14,15). Briefly, 2 mg TXDK were
incubated with 15 mg histamine dichloride (Merck,Darmstadt), to
which 10 μCi ^{3}H-histamine (New England Nuclear Co., Dreieichen-
hain, spec.act. 6.1 Ci/mmole) had been added, and 15 mg of 1-
ethyl-3-(3-dimethylaminopropyl)carbodiimide hydrochloride (Ott
Chemical Co., Muskegon, USA) in a total volume of 2.5 ml (5%
ethanol). The pH was adjusted to 5.5 and incubation was carried
out at room temperature overnight. The various compounds in the
incubate were then separated by thin layer chromatography (n-
butanol-acetic acid-H_2O 75:10:25, by vol.). The TXDK-histamine
conjugate (Rf 0.35) was scraped off and eluted with 10% aqueous
methanol. An aliquot of the conjugate (5 μg) was iodinated with
^{125}I using the chloramine-T method (16). $Na^{125}I$, 10 μl (500 μCi),
was added to 50 μl sodium phosphate buffer, pH 7.4, and 50 μl of
TXDK-histamine solution. Then 5 μl (5 μg) chloramine T was added
and the reaction stopped after 40 seconds by the addition of
5 μl (32.5 μg) sodium metabisulfite. The products of the reaction
were purified immediately by thin layer chromatography as described by Maclouf et al. (14) and tested for binding to the anti-
TXDK antiplasma.

2.   Radioimmunoassay:
          Radioimmunoassay of TXDK in 20 μl aliquots of guinea
pig plasma was performed as described previously for determination of 15-keto-13,14-dihydro-$PGF_{2\alpha}$ and 6-keto-$PGF_{1\alpha}$ in plasma
(17), except that incubations were not carried out at 37°C, but
at 4°C. Goat anti-rabbit- ɣ -globulin (Calbiochem-Behring,Gies-
sen) was added after 2 hours and incubated overnight to separate
·free and antibody-bound fractions of label. The preparation of
the anti-TXDK antiplasma used (final dilution in the assay
1: 80 000) has been described previously (13).

3.   Extraction and thin layer chromatography:
          Extraction of acidified (pH 3.2) guinea pig plasma with
ethyl acetate and thin layer chromatography (solvent systems:
diethyl ether-methanol-acetic acid 90:1:2, by vol., and chloro-
form-H_2O-methanol-acetic acid 90:0.8:8:1, by vol.) followed by
radioimmunoassay of TXDK of eluted zones were performed as
described previously for organ perfusates (13).

4.   Animal experiments:
          Guinea pigs of either sex (400-900 g) were anaestheti-

zed with urethane (1.2 g/kg i.p.) and received heparin (1 000 U
i.p./animal) and gallamine (1 mg/kg i.p.). Some of the animals
had been sensitized with ovalbumin as described previously (12).
The trachea, arteria carotis dextra and vena jugularis externa
were cannulated. The animals were respired with a positive
pressure pump (Braun,Melsungen). After an equilibration period
of at least 15 min bronchospasm was elicited in sensitized guinea pigs by i.v. injection of ovalbumin (10 mg/kg) and in non-
sensitized animals by i.v. injection of histamine dichloride
(50 µg base/kg). Blood (250 µl) was collected on ice from the
arteria carotis into 50 µl indomethacin solution (1 mg/ml, dissolved in 0.1M sodium phosphate buffer, pH 7.4) 10 and 2 min
before and 0.5, 2 and 5 min after injection of ovalbumin or
histamine respectively. The plasma was rapidly separated from
blood cells by centrifugation at 4°C (1 500xg, 10 min) and stored frozen until analyzed by radioimmunoassay for TXDK.

Results and Discussion

The use of the monovalent iodinated tracer instead of
a polyvalent tracer (13) improved, as expected, the sensitivity
of the radioimmunoassay for TXDK more than 20 fold, 18pg causing
10% inhibition of binding of label to the antiplasma. The radioimmunoassay is highly specific, the only compound cross-reacting
at 100 ng being 15-keto-13,14-dihydro-PGF$_{2\alpha}$ (29% inhibition of
binding of label to the anti-TXDK antiplasma). The great sensitivity of the radioimmunoassay allowed the quantitative determination of TXDK in small aliquots (20 µl) of guinea pig plasma
samples. The accuracy of the TXDK determination in guinea pig
plasma is shown in fig. 1. Larger volumes of guinea pig plasma
could not be analyzed, since they interfered non-specifically
with the radioimmunoassay.

In some preliminary in vivo experiments plasma levels
of immunoreactive TXDK during anaphylactic shock and after histamine injection (50 µg/kg i.v.) were determined. While the normal
plasma levels of TXDK in sensitized and non-sensitized guinea
pigs were below or close to the detection limit of the radioimmunoassay (900 pg/ml), a large increase was observed after antigen
injection into sensitized animals. TXDK levels rose to 14.4 ±
10.4 ng/ml at 0.5 min, 126.9 ± 99.6 ng/ml at 2 min and 208.4 ±
149.2 ng/ml at 5 min after challenge (means ± S.E.M., n=3).After
the injection of histamine into non-sensitized guinea pigs the
following plasma levels of immunoreactive TXDK were found: 5.9 ±
1.3 ng/ml at 0.5 min, 4.8 ± 0.7 ng/ml at 2 min and 4.6 ± 0.3 ng/
ml at 5 min (means ± S.E.M., n=3). The immunoreactive TXDK found
in guinea pig plasma during anaphylactic shock was further cha-
racterized by thin layer chromatography. It was found that the
immunoreactive material co-chromatographed with authentic TXDK
in two different solvent systems.

Our results show that similar to the findings with
isolated perfused sensitized guinea pig lungs after challenge
(10,13) large amounts of TXDK are released during anaphylactic

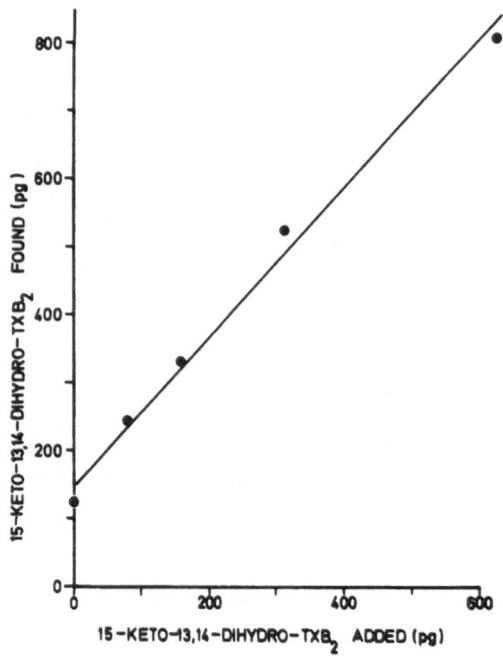

Fig. 1   Accuracy of the radioimmunoassay for TXDK. Known
amounts of TXDK were added to 20 µl aliquots of a plasma sample
obtained from a sensitized guinea pig 30 seconds after challenge.

shock in vivo. Obviously a significant fraction of the total
TXA_2 and/or TXB_2 synthesized by anaphylactic guinea pig lungs is
metabolized within the lungs before being released. Histamine,
which is also released from anaphylactic guinea pig lungs (2)
and releases TXA_2 from guinea pig lung tissue in vitro (3) might
contribute to the elevated TXDK plasma levels observed in anaphylactic shock in vivo.

        Radioimmunological determination of TXDK in plasma
might be a more reliable method than TXB_2 determination (9) to
study TX release by drugs and especially during anaphylactic
shock of guinea pigs in vivo. Roberts et al. (18,19) have investigated the metabolism of TXB_2 in man and monkey. They found
substantial formation of 15-keto-13,14-dihydro-derivatives of
TXB_2 after initial dehydrogenation of the hemiacetal alcohol

group at C-11. From the present results it seems possible that determination of plasma levels of such compounds might be useful for the study of endogenous TX synthesis in man.

Acknowledgement

We thank Dr. F.A. Fitzpatrick and Dr. J. Pike, Upjohn Co., Kalamazoo, USA for the gift of 15-keto-13,14-dihydro-TXB$_2$ and PGs. This work was supported by the Deutsche Forschungs-gemeinschaft.

References

1.   M. Hamberg, J. Svensson and B. Samuelsson, Thromboxanes: a new group of biologically active compounds derived from prostaglandin endoperoxides, Proc.Natl.Acad.Sci.USA 72, 2994-2998 (1975).

2.   P.J. Piper and J.R. Vane, Release of additional factors in anaphylaxis and its antagonism by anti-inflammatory drugs, Nature 223, 29-35 (1969).

3.   R.J. Gryglewski, Generation of prostaglandin and thrombox-ane-like substances by large airways and lung parenchyma, in: Prostaglandins and Thromboxanes (Eds. F. Berti, B. Samuelsson and G.P. Velo, Plenum Press, New York and London, 1977).

4.   E. Granström, H. Kindahl and B. Samuelsson, Radioimmuno-assay for thromboxane B$_2$, Anal. Lett. 9, 611-627 (1976).

5.   H. Anhut, W. Bernauer and B.A. Peskar, Radioimmunological determination of thromboxane release in cardiac anaphy-laxis, Europ. J. Pharmacol. 44, 85-88 (1977).

6.   H. Sors, P. Pradelles and F. Dray, Analytical methods for thromboxane B$_2$ measurement and validation of radioimmuno-assay by gas liquid chromatography-mass spectrometry, Prostaglandins 16, 277-290 (1978).

7.   F.A. Fitzpatrick and R.R. Gorman, Platelet rich plasma transforms exogenous prostaglandin endoperoxide H$_2$ into thromboxane A$_2$, Prostaglandins 14, 881-889 (1977).

8.   J. Maclouf, H. Kindahl, E. Granström and B. Samuelsson, Thromboxane A$_2$ and prostaglandin endoperoxide H$_2$ form covalently linked derivatives with human serum albumin, Abstract, Fourth Int. Prostaglandin Conference, Washington D.C. 1979, p. 73.

9.   E. Granström, Radioimmunoassay of prostaglandins, Prosta-glandins 15, 3-17 (1978).

10. W. Dawson, J.R. Boot, A.F. Cockerill, D.N.B. Mallen and
     D.J. Osborne, Release of novel prostaglandins and thrombox-
     anes after immunological challenge of guinea pig lung,
     Nature 262, 699-702 (1976).

11. A.A. Mathé and L. Levine, Release of prostaglandins and
     metabolites from guinea pig lung: inhibition by catechol-
     amines, Prostaglandins 4, 877-890 (1973).

12. R.Liebig, W. Bernauer and B.A. Peskar, Release of prosta-
     glandins, a prostaglandin metabolite, slow-reacting sub-
     stance and histamine from anaphylactic lungs and its modi-
     fication by catecholamines, Naunyn-Schmiedeberg's Arch.
     Pharmacol. 284, 279-293 (1974).

13. H. Anhut, B.A. Peskar and W. Bernauer, Release of 15-keto-
     13,14-dihydro-thromboxane B_2 and prostaglandin D_2 during
     anaphylaxis as measured by radioimmunoassay, Naunyn-
     Schmiedeberg's Arch. Pharmacol. 305, 247-252 (1978).

14. J. Maclouf, M. Pradel, P. Pradelles and F. Dray, ^{125}I deri-
     vatives of prostaglandins, a novel approach in prosta-
     glandin analysis by radioimmunoassay, Biochim. Biophys.
     Acta 431, 139-146 (1976).

15. H. Sors, J. Maclouf, P. Pradelles and F. Dray, The use of
     iodinated tracers for a sensitive radioimmunoassay of 13,
     14-dihydro-15-keto-prostaglandin F_α, Biochim. Biophys.
     Acta 486, 553-564 (1977).

16. F.C. Greenwood, W.M. Hunter and J.S. Glover, The pre-
     paration of I^{131} labelled human growth hormone of high
     specific radioactivity, Biochem. J. 89, 114-123 (1963).

17. B.A Peskar, Ch. Steffens and B.M. Peskar, Radioimmuno-
     assay of 6-keto-prostaglandin $F_{1\alpha}$ in biological material,
     in: Radioimmunoassay of drugs and hormones (Eds. A.Alber-
     tini, M. DaPrada and B.A. Peskar, North Holland Publ. Co.,
     in press).

18. L.J. Roberts II, B.J. Sweetman and J.A. Oates, Metabolism
     of thromboxane B_2 in man, Abstract Nr. 2010, 7th Int.
     Congress of Pharmacol., Paris 1978.

19. L.J. Roberts II, B.J. Sweetman and J.A. Oates, Metabolism
     of thromboxane B_2 in the monkey, J. Biol. Chem. 253, 5305-
     5318 (1978).

Chapter Two

PROSTAGLANDINS AS MEDIATORS OF ACUTE
INFLAMMATION AND PAIN

PROSTAGLANDINS AS MEDIATORS OF INFLAMMATION - VASCULAR ASPECTS

J. Westwick
Thrombosis Research Unit, Rayne Institute, King's College Hospital,
London SE5.

Oedema is an important aspect of acute inflammation. Oedema is thought to
be the result of an increase in vascular permeability of capillaries and post
capillary venules to plasma proteins (1) with or without a concomitant
increase in blood flow.

In this paper I would like to present evidence concerning the possible roles
of prostaglandins (PGs) in the vasodilation and the increase in vascular
permeability of an inflammatory reaction. Both microscopic and isotopic
techniques have been used to examine the microvascular effects of prostaglandins.

Vasodilation

The classical method of studying vasodilation is the direct microscopic
observation of arterioles and venules of a microvascular bed, an example of
this is the hamster cheek pouch preparation (2). It is the tone of the
precapillary arterioles, which control the blood flow through any organ.
They are both innervated and sensitive to blood bourne agents and are capable
of remarkable changes in diameter. Thus they can dramatically change local
blood flow by vasodilation or intense vasoconstriction. The diameter of
such arterioles can be constantly monitored by projecting the image of an
arteriole onto a photocell. A pen recorder trace of the vessel diameter in
microns can be produced after calibration of the photocell output (3).

Using this technique the relative potency of the classical prostaglandins have
been determined by infusing the compounds into the Krebs solution bathing the
cheek pouch membrane (3). The order of potency was found to be as follows
PGE_2 {1.2} > 13, 14 dihydro - PGE_2 {6} > PGE_1 {8} > 15 - keto - PGE_2 {380},
the figure in parenthesis is the concentration in ng required to produce a
50% vasodilation in noradrenaline constricted arterioles.

These experiments demonstrated that loss of the 15 - OH group from the E
series PGs produced a 300 fold loss in potency. Also, the presence of the
13, 14 double bond was not essential for vasodilator activity. In this
experimental model $PGF_{2\alpha}$ was inactive and PGD_2 was a vasoconstrictor.

Thus PGs of the E type, which do not have a 15 - keto groups are potent
vasodilators, not only in the hamster but also in human skin (4, 5) guinea-
pig skin (6, 7), rat skin (8), rabbit skin (9) and dog synovial microcirculation (10). In all the aforementioned examples the E type PG were active
at ng concentrations at producing a vasodilation. Similar or higher concentrations of the PGs of the E type have been detected in a variety of
inflammatory exudates such as human burn blister fluid (11), scalded tissue
(12), and synovial fluid from arthritic joints (13). Thus there is good

agreement concerning the amount of E type PG produced in an inflammatory
condition and the amount necessary to produce a vasodilation.

A common precursor of the 2 series PGs, thromboxanes and prostacyclin (PGI_2)
is the unstable endoperoxide, PGG_2. The effect of PGG_2 on arterioles has
been examined in the hamster cheek pouch preparation (14). The effect on
arterioles was dependent on the concentration of PGG_2 and on the tone of the
vessel. In arterioles with a resting tone, low concentrations (2-5ngs) of
PGG_2 produced a vasodilation only. Higher concentration (25 - 200ng)
produced a transient vasoconstriction followed by a protracted phase of
vasodilatation. In arterioles without a resting tone high concentrations
(25 to 100ngs) produced a transient vasoconstriction only. Both the vasoconstrictor and vasodilator actions of PGG_2 demonstrated tachyphylaxis in
the hamster cheek pouch preparation. The biphasic action of PGG_2 on blood
flow was also demonstrated in rabbit skin (14). We concluded from these
studies that if these observations could be extrapolated to conditions
where vascular injury occurs, it seemed unlikely because of its acute and
tachyphylactic nature that PGG_2 could be responsible for protracted periods
of vasoconstriction.

However the PGG_2 could be responsible for acute periods of constriction as
are often observed in response to injurious stimuli. The protracted phase
of vasodilation observed with PGG_2 may be produced by enzymic or non
enzymic products of PGG_2.

A likely candidate, to be the enzymic product is PGI_2, which is known to be
formed by vessel walls from PGG_2 (15). Indeed PGI_2 has been shown to be a
potent vasodilator in rats, rabbits (16, 17), hamster (18), and man (5).
There is also increasing evidence to suggest that PGI_2 is produced in
inflammatory conditions for example in granuloma tissue (19), and in macrophage tissue culture (20).

Because of the advances in PG research, it may be necessary to repeat the
experiments in which E series PGs were detected in inflammatory conditions
to determine if other endoperoxide metabolites were produced, such as
thromboxane B_2 and 6 - oxo - $PGF_{1\alpha}$. At this stage it is not possible to say
with any certainty whether PGE_2 or PGI_2 is the PG responsible for the vasodilator effect at the site of inflammation.

Increased Vascular Permeability

To determine the effects of PGs on vascular permeability to macromolecules a
variety of techniques have been employed. The validity of the results is
dependent upon the suitability of the technique employed to measure increased
vascular permeability. That is plasma exudation can result from an increase
in intra-luminal hydrostatic pressure with only a small change in increased
vascular permeability. The relationship between exudation and blood flow
has been discussed by Williams and Peck (20).

Vascular permeability has been measured by observing the extravasation of
intravenously injected dyes such as Evans blue and pontamine blue. These
dyes bind to plasma proteins, in particular albumin but as the degree of
binding is unknown it is difficult to interpret the results (21). This
variability has been overcome by either using fluorescein labelled dextrans

or $\{^{131}I\}$ human serum albumin which have defined molecular weight and chemical stability (22, 6).

In rat skin, PGE_1 and PGE_2 produced an increase in dye extravasation (22,23). Also in the hamster cheek pouch PGE_1 and PGE_2 increased the number of leakage sites at the post capillary venule measured as the extravasation of fluorescein labelled dextran (24). On human skin (4, 18) PGE_1, PGE_2 and PGI_2 induced erythema without oedema. However oedema was reported in 2 out of 5 subjects following PGE_1 or PGE_2 injection into forearm skin (23). PGs were ineffective at increasing vascular permeability in the guinea-pig and rabbit skin (6,9,14,17) but were found to be partially effective by other workers (25).

Although there is some dispute as to whether PGs per se increase vascular permeability, there is no doubt that PGs, in particular PGE_1, PGE_2 and PGI_2 potentiate the exudation induced by agents such as histamine and bradykinin (6-9. 14, 17, 20, 23-25).

REFERENCES

1. MAJNO, G and PALADE, G.E. Studies on inflammation. I. The effect of histamine and serotonin on vascular permeability. An electron microscopic study. J. Biophys. Biochem. Cytol. 11, 571-605 (1961).

2. DULING, B.R. The preparation and use of the hamster cheek pouch for studies of the microcirculation. Microvasc. Res. 5, 423-429 (1973).

3. WESTWICK, J. and LEWIS, G.P. Reversal of noradrenaline-induced constriction of hamster cheek pouch arterioles by prostaglandins and their metabolites. Bibl. Anat. 16, 466-469 (1977).

4. JUHLIN, L and MICHAELSSON, G. Cutaneous vascular reactions to prostaglandins in healthy subjects and in patients with urticaria and atopic dermatitis. Acta. derm. venereol. (Stockh) 49, 251-261 (1969).

5. HIGGS, E.A. O'GRADY, J., THROWER, P.A. and MONCADA, S. Prostacyclin: inflammation effects in human skin. In Abstracts Fourth International Prostaglandin Conference, Washington, D.C. May 27-31st, (1979) p 48.

6. WILLIAMS, T.J. and MORLEY,J. Prostaglandins as potentiators of increased vascular permeability in inflammation. Nature, Lond. 246, 215-217 (1973).

7. JOHNSTON, M.G., HAY, J.B. and MOVAT, H.Z. The modulation of enhanced vascular permeability by prostaglandins through alterations in blood flow. Agents and Action 6, 705-711 (1976).

8. MONCADA, S., FERREIRA, S.H. and VANE, J.R. Prostaglandins, aspirin-like drugs and the oedema of inflammation. Nature, Lond. 246, 217-219 (1973).

9.   WILLIAMS, T.J. The pro-inflammatory activity of E-, A-, D- and F- type
     prostaglandins and analogues 16, 16 dimethyl - PGE_2 and (15S)-15-methyl
     -PGE_2 in rabbit skin; the relationship between potentiation of plasma
     exudation and local blood flow changes. Br. J. Pharmac. 56, 341-343P

10. DICK, W.C., GRENNAN, D.M. and ZEITLIN, I.J. Studies on the relative
     effects of prostaglandins, bradykinin, 5-hydroxytryptamine and hista-
     mine on the synovial microcirculation in dogs. Br. J. Pharmac, 56,
     313-316, (1976).

11. ARTURSON, G., HAMBERG, M. and JONSSON, C.E. Prostaglandins in human
     burn blister fluid. Acta. Physiol. scand. 87, 270-276 (1973).

12. ANGGARD, E. and JONSSON, G.E. Efflux of prostaglandins from scalded
     tissue. Acta. Physiol. scand. 81, 440-447 (1971).

13. BLACKHAM, A, FARMER, J.B., RADZIWONIK, H. and WESTWICK, J. The role
     of prostaglandins in rabbit mono-articular arthritis. Br. J. Pharmac.
     51, 35-44. (1974).

14. LEWIS, G.P., WESTWICK, J. and WILLIAMS, T.J. Microvascular responses
     produced by the prostaglandin endoperoxide PGG_2 in vivo. Br. J.
     Pharmac. 59, 442P   (1977)

15. MONCADA, S., GRYGLEWSKI, R., BUNTING, S. and VANE, J.R. An enzyme
     isolated from arteries transforms prostaglandin endoperoxides to an
     unstable substance that inhibits aggregation. Nature, Lond. 263
     663-667 (1976)

16. ARMSTRONG, J.M., LATTIMER, N., MONCADA, S. and VANE, J.R. Comparison of
     the vasodepressor effects of prostacyclin and 6-oxo-prostaglandin $F_{1\alpha}$
     with those of prostaglandin E_2 in rats and rabbits. Br. J. Pharmac.
     62, 125-130 (1978).

17. WILLIAMS, T.J. Prostaglandin E_2, prostaglandin I_2 and the vascular
     changes of inflammation. Br. J. Pharmac. 65, 517-524 (1979).

18. HIGGS, H.A., MONCADA, S. and VANE, J.R. Prostacyclin is a potent
     dilator of arterioles in the hamster cheek pouch. J. Physiol. 275,
     30-31P (1978).

19. CHANG, W.C. MUROTA, S., MATSUO, M. and TSURUFUJI, S. A new prostaglandin
     transformed from arachidonic acid in carrageenin-induced granuloma.
     Biochem. Biophys. Res. Commun. 72, 1259-1264 (1976)

20. WILLIAMS, T.J. and PECK, M.J. Role of prostaglandin mediated vaso-
     dilation in inflammation. Nature. Lond. 270, 530-532 (1977).

21. LEVICK, J.R. and MICHEL, C.C. The permeability of individually
     perfused frog mesenteric capillaries to Tl^{824} and T1824 albumin as
     evidence for a large pore system. Quart. J. Exp. Physiol. 58,
     67-85 (1973).

22. KALEY, G. and WEINER, R. Microcirculatory studies with prostaglandin
     E_1, In Prostaglandin Symposium of the Worcester Foundation for
     Experimental Biology ed. Ramwell, P.W. and Shaw, J.E. pp321-328.
     New York: Intersciences Publishers (1968).

23. CRUNKHORN, P. and WILLIS, A.L. Cutaneous reactions to intradermal
     prostaglandins. Br. J. Pharmac. 41, 49-56 (1971).

24. SVENSJO, E. Bradykinin and prostaglandin E_1 E_2 and $F_{2\alpha}$-induced
     macromolecular leakage in the hamster cheek pouch. Prostaglandins and
     Medicine 1, 397-410 (1978).

25. IKEDA, K., TANAKA, K., KATORI, M. Potentiation of bradykinin-induced
     vascular permeability increase by prostaglandin E_2 and arachidonic
     acid in rabbit skin. Prostaglandins, 10, 747-758 (1975).

EFFECTS OF PROSTAGLANDINS ON PERIPHERAL NOCICEPTORS IN ACUTE
INFLAMMATION

M B Tyers and Hazel Haywood

ABSTRACT

        The effects of different prostaglandins were deter-
mined on (a) the hyperalgesia produced by subplantar injections of yeast given into the hind paws of weanling rats, and
(b) the reflex vasopressor responses to bradykinin (BK)
injected dose-arterially into the spleen of anaesthetised
cats and dogs. In the rat prostaglandins ($E_1>E_2>> F_{2\alpha} =
F_{2\beta}=A_2=D_2=I_2=0$) injected into the same paw either with the
yeast or 25min later reduced the latency to the onset of
hyperalgesia. In the cat and dog prostaglandins ($E_1>E_2>F_{2\alpha}
>F_{2\beta}>A_1=A_2=0$) potentiated vasopressor responses to BK and
reversed the inhitibion of BK responses by indomethacin.
It is likely that prostaglandins sensitize peripheral
nociceptors through a specific prostaglandin receptor.

INTRODUCTION

        The mediation of pain associated with acute
inflammation is attributed to the release of chemical
substances that stimulate peripheral nociceptors. Many
substances that are released in acute inflammation[1],
such as bradykinin (BK), histamine and 5-hydroxytryptamine

(5HT) when injected close-arterially into the spleen of dogs [2,3] cause a 'pseudo-affective' response characterised by vocalisation, biting, struggling and a reflex rise in blood pressure [4]. Bradykinin injected into the splenic artery in an isolated perfused dog spleen preparation causes the release of prostaglandins which are detectable in the venous outflow [5,6]. Aspirin-like analgesic drugs inhibit both the pseudo-affective response and the prostaglandin production induced by bradykinin. Prosta-glandins E_2 and $F_{2\alpha}$ are also released during an acute inflammatory response. The mechanism of the analgesic action of the peripherally-acting aspirin-like drugs is most likely due to their inhibitory action on prosta-glandin synthesis [7,8].

Prostaglandins injected intra-arterially, subdermally or applied directly to a blister base cause little or no pain [9-11]. But when injected intra-arterially into the spleen of dogs E-prostaglandins cause long-lasting sensitization of peripheral nociceptors to algesic agents [5,8]. The nociceptor sensitizing action of prostaglandins has also been reported in other experimen-tal pain models in anaesthetised animals [12-14].

The present experiments were carried out to determine the effects of different prostaglandins (a) on the development of hyperalgesia to subplantar injections of yeast given into the hind paws of conscious rats, and (b) in potentiating the reflex vasopressor responses to intrasplenic injections of bradykinin and reversing the block of the responses by indomethacin in the anaesthetized cat and dog.

METHODS

Effects on yeast-induced hyperalgesia in the rat

The effects of prostaglandins E_1, E_2, $F_{2\alpha}$, $F_{2\beta}$, A_2, D_2, I_2 and arachidonic acid on the development of hyperalgesia to subplantar yeast injections in the hind paws of rats were determined. Tests were carried out in dose-

groups of 6 rats (male, AH random-bred hooded, 35-80g).
Data were accumulated from duplicated tests carried out on
3 separate days such that final dose-groups comprised 18
rats. To eliminate cage interaction the rats were randomised
according to treatment such that each cage contained animals
receiving different treatments. Animals and test solutions
were colour-coded such that the operators were not aware of
the treatments the rats were receiving.

      Nociceptive pressure thresholds for the right hind
paw of each rat were determined using an 'Analgesymeter'
(Ugo Basile, Milan). The nociceptive response was usually
a shrill vocalisation or a strong attempt to withdraw the
paw. Each rat then received an injection of 0.1ml of 5% $^{W}/v$
suspension of Brewer's yeast (CWE Ltd., Cawston, Norfolk) in
saline given subcutaneously into the subplantar surface of
the right hind paw and then returned to their cages.
Prostaglandins (see DRUGS) were either mixed and injected
with, or given 25min after the yeast injection. Nociceptive
pressure thresholds were redetermined at 30, 60, 120, 180 and
240 min. after yeast injections.

Effects on responses to intrasplenic
bradykinin in the cat and dog

      Cats (1.9 -4.4kg) and Beagle dogs (7.1 -10.3kg) of
either sex were anaesthetised with halothane (3.5% in $N_2O:O_2$)
or thiopentone respectively and maintained on chloralose,
75mg/kg iv. The femoral vein and artery were cannulated for
drug administrations and recordings of blood pressure respect-
ively.The spleen was exposed through a mid-line incision in
the abdomen. A small branch of the splenic artery was cannulated with pp10 tubing for retrograde intra-arterial injections; 2 cannulae were inserted into the same branch artery so
that bolus injections of bradykinin could be given without
disturbing infusions of prostaglandins.

      Dose-response curves were obtained for the reflex
vasopressor response induced by dose-arterial injections of
BK, 0.2-10µg, into the spleen. Doses of BK were given at
10-15min intervals. To determine the effects of prosta-
glandins A_1, A_2, E_1, E_2, $F_{2\alpha}$ and $F_{2\beta}$ on the reflex vasopressor
responses solutions of prostaglandins were infused at a
constant rate of 0.5ml/min for 1min immediately before inject-

ion of BK. The minimum effective dose was determined for
each prostaglandin to (a) potentiate responses to BK, and (b)
to reverse the block of BK responses caused by indomethacin,
3mg/kg iv.

DRUGS

        The following compounds have been used:
Brewers yeast (CWE Ltd., Cawston, Norfolk), indomethacin
(Sigma Chem. Co.Ltd.); Prostaglandins E_1, E_2, $F_{2\beta}$, A_1 and
A_2 (Ono Pharmaceuticals, Japan); $PGF_{2\alpha}$ (dinoprost
trimethamine, UpJohn); PGI_2 and PGD_2 were synthesized
in the Chemistry Research Dept., Glaxo Group Research Ltd.,
Ware. PGI_2 was dissolved in Tris HCl pH9 and diluted as
required in Tris buffer pH8. All other prostaglandins were
dissolved in 1% sodium bicarbonate and diluted in normal
saline.

RESULTS

        Effects on yeast-induced hyperalgesia in the rat

        Subplantar injections of a yeast suspension into
the hind paws of rats caused characteristic biphasic effects
on nociceptive pressure thresholds [15]. Initially there
was an increase in threshold which developed at the same rate
as the increase in paw volume. After about 60min.the thresholds started to decrease towards normal and reached a steady
level of hyperalgesia about 4h after yeast. Prostaglandin E_1,
0.01-1.0µg, injected at the same time as the yeast, reduced
the initial increase in threshold and, at the higher doses,
hyperalgesia had already developed at the 30min. reading
(Fig.1). The maximum hyperalgesia achieved at 4h after yeast
was unchanged by PGE_1. PGE_2, 0.01-1.0µg reduced the
initial hypoalgesic phase of yeast injection but nociceptive
thresholds were only reduced back to pre-yeast values (Fig.1).

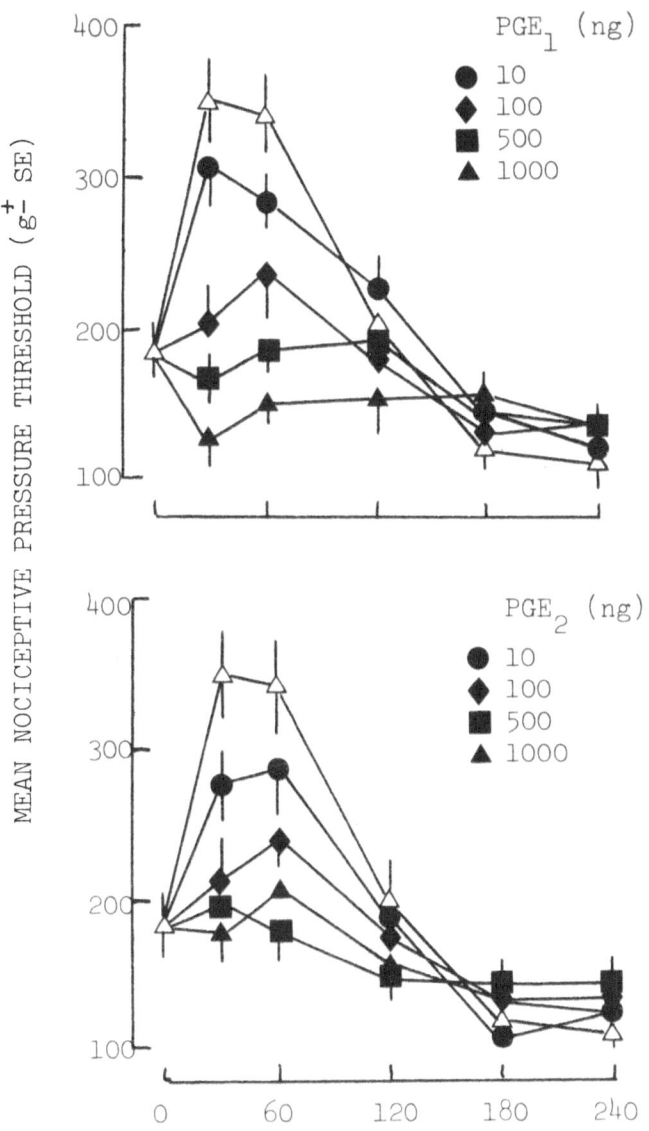

TIME AFTER SUBPLANTAR INJECTION (min)

Fig. 1.   Effects of prostaglandins E_1 and E_2, 10-1000ng, on changes in nociceptive pressure thresholds induced by sub-plantar injections of yeast in the rat hind paw.
($\triangle$) = yeast alone.

Thus, unlike for PGE_1, the onset time to hyperalgesia, ie.
the time from yeast injection until the first significant
reduction in thresholds below pre-yeast values, was not
significantly reduced by PGE_2. PGE_2 was also slightly
less potent than PGE_1 but dose-response curves were not
parallel (Fig 2). Neither prostaglandin affected the
development of oedema (Fig.3). Arachidonic acid, 100µg,
reduced the initial hypoalgesia when injected with the yeast
but PGA_2, $F_{2\alpha}$, $F_{2\beta}$, D_2 and I_2, all at 0.5µg, had no
effect on yeast-induced changes in nociceptive pressure
thresholds. In some further experiments either PGE_1,
0.0025-0.1µg or PGI_2, 0.004-0.5µg was injected into the paw
at 25min after the yeast injections. At this time PGE_1
was more potent than when it was injected with the yeast
and caused at 3-fold shift of the dose-response curve to the
left (Fig.2). PGI_2 was inactive.

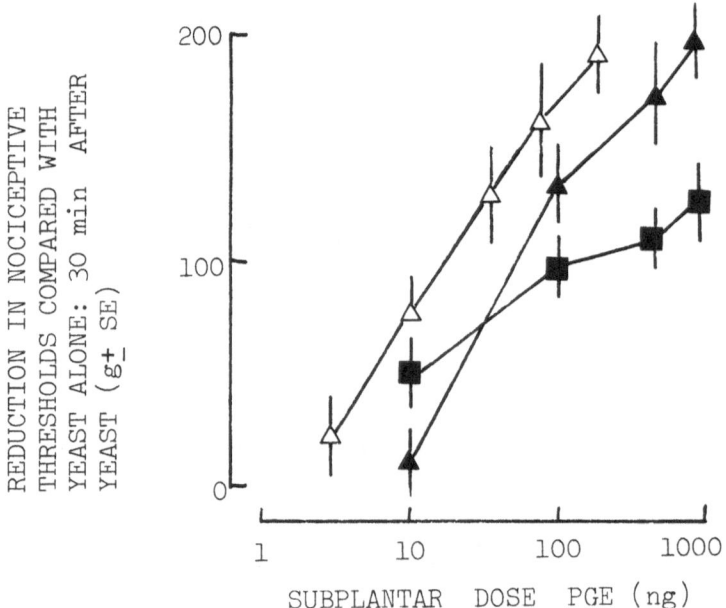

Fig. 2. Effects of prostaglandin E_1 (▲△) and E_2 (■) on
nociceptive pressure thresholds 30 min after yeast injection
into the rat hind paw. Prostaglandins were either given
with the yeast (closed symbols) or 25 min after the yeast
(open symbols).

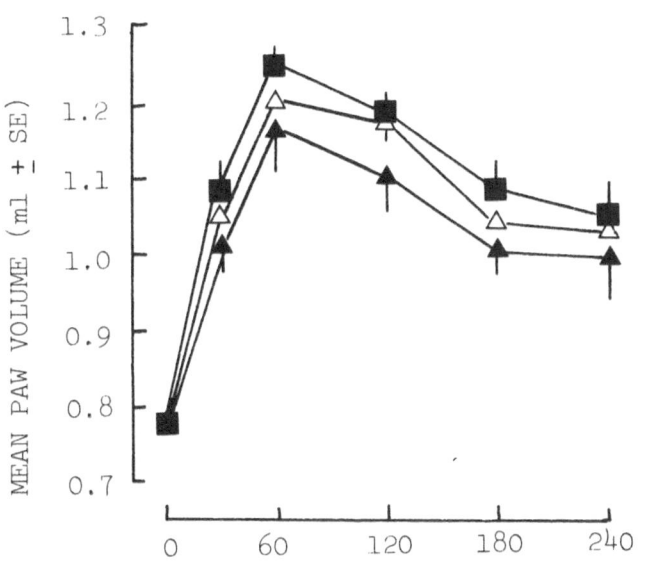

Fig 3.   Effects of prostaglandins E_1 (▲) and E_2 (■)
500ng on yeast-induced oedema in the rat hind paw.
(△) = yeast alone

Effects on responses to intraplenic
bradykinin in the cat and dog.

In both the anaesthetised cat and dog close-arterial
injections of BK, 0.2-10µg given into the splenic arterial
cannula, caused dose-related reflex vasopressor responses of
3-45 mmHg.   The responses occurred after a latency of about
20s and lasted for 1-2min. In each experiment the dose of BK
was selected to give a response of 50-75% maximum.   This was
usually within the range 0.5-2µg.   To determine the effects of
prostaglandins 3 control responses to BK were first obtained.
Prostaglandins were then slowly infused for 1min immediately

prior to the next BK injection. BK, without infusions of
prostaglandins, was given at 10min intervals thereafter until
the vasopressor responses returned to control levels. In the
cat, PGE_1, 0.005-0.04µg/kg, and PGE_2, 0.03-0.2µg/kg given
in this manner, caused dose-dependent potentiations of the
vasopressor responses to BK. Responses returned to normal
within 30-40min after PG infusion. Responses were usually
potentiated to a level about equal to the predetermined
maximum effect of BK. On occasion the higher doses of PGE_1
and PGE_2 potentiated the BK response beyond the original
maximum by up to 60%. This latter effect was probably due
to a lightening of the anaesthesia; the depth of chloralose
anaesthesia is critical in these experiments. In 3 of our 6
cats tested $PGF_{2\alpha}$, 0.2-1.0 µg/kg, and $PGF_{2\beta}$, 0.32-1.0µg/kg,
potentiations of the vasopressor responses but were less potent
than PGE_1. The reason for this variation between animals
was not clear and was not related to age, sex or depth of
anaesthesia. PGA_1 and PGA_2, 1µg/kg, were inactive. In
the dog PGE_1, 0.0025- 0.02µg/kg, PGE_2, 0.1-0. 8 µg/kg, $PGF_{2\alpha}$,
0.16-0.64, and $PGF_{2\beta}$, 0.16-0.64µg/kg were all slightly more
potent potentiators of BK than in the cat but the rank order
and potency ratios were very similar in the two species.
$PGF_{2\alpha}$ and $F_{2\beta}$ again were effective in only 4 out of 6
dogs tested. The minimum effective potentiating doses of the
prostaglandins tested in the cat and dog are given in Table 1.
None of the prostaglandins given alone close-arterially to
the spleen produced any apparent stimulation of nociceptors.
        In further experiments in the cat BK responses were
greatly reduced (75-95%) by indomethacin, 3mg/kg iv. In these
animals close-arterial infusions of PGE_1, 0.01-0.1µg/kg,
PGE_2, 0.06-0.24 µg/kg and $PGF_{2\alpha}$, 0.16-0.64µg/kg for 1 min
prior to BK injections restored the reflex vasopressor responses. When the infusions of prostaglandins were then
stopped the responses to BK gradually diminished again.
Close-arterial infusions of PGA_1, 0.64µg/kg, did not reverse
the inhibition of BK responses caused by indomethacin.

TABLE 1   Minimum effective doses of prostaglandins that
            cause potentiation of reflex vasopressor
            responses to intrasplenic injections of BK in the
            anaesthetised cat and dog.

Species	Minimum effective dose (ng/kg ia) mean of n experiments					
	PGE$_1$	PGE$_2$	PGF$_{2\alpha}$	PGF$_{2\beta}$	PGA$_1$	PGA$_2$
Cat	5	30	200	320	Inactive at 1000	Inactive at 1000
(n)	(3)	(3)	(3)	(3)	(2)	(2)
Dog	2.5	10	160	160	1000	Not tested
(n)	(3)	(3)	(4)	(4)	(2)	(2)

DISCUSSION

        For a substance to be considered as a mediator of
pain in acute inflammation it must conform to certain
criteria. First, the substance(s) must be shown to be
released at some phase during an inflammatory attack;
second, the substance(s) should produce or play an essential
part in the stimulation of peripheral nociceptors, and third,
inhibition of the formation, release or action of the sub-
stance(s) should produce analgesia, or conversely, an
increase in these should cause hyperalgesia.
        Of the substances released and detected in
inflammatory exudates the most prominent in the early
phases of acute inflammation are histamine, 5-hydroxy-
tryptamine, bradykinin and prostaglandins E$_2$ and F$_{2\alpha}$
[1,16]. The first three of these substances, but not
PGE$_2$ or F$_{2\alpha}$, stimulate peripheral nociceptors in the cat
and dog spleen[3], dog heart[13] dog knee joint[12] and
in the vasoisolated perfused rabbit ear[14]. The results
obtained in the present study in the anaesthetised cat and

dog and in the conscious rat confirm previous studies
showing that prostaglandins E_1 and E_2, and to a less
extent $PGF_{2\alpha}$, sensitize peripheral nociceptors to these
algesic agents. PGE_1 is undoubtedly the most potent of
the PG's tested but there is no evidence that it occurs
naturally in inflammatory exudates. It is more likely
that PGE_2 is the natural mediator of inflammatory pain.

From the experiments on the mediators of carageenin-
induced acute inflammation there appear to be three distinct
phases following activation of complement[1]. There is
an initial phase in which histamine and 5-hydroxytryptamine
are released, a second phase commences some 30-60min later
and is mediated by kinins, and soon after this a third phase
is mediated by prostaglandins. The hyperalgesia following
subplantar injections of either carageenin[15] or yeast
into the hind paws of rats does not appear for 60-90min
and reaches a maximum at about 4h. Therefore, the first
appearance of hyperalgesia is at about the same time as the
onset of the second phase of inflammation and reaches a
maximum well after commencement of the prostaglandin (third)
phase. The degree of hyperalgesia appears to be related
to the relative concentrations of bradykinin and prostaglandins at the inflammatory site. This has been shown
experimentally in pain models such as the dog spleen and perfused rabbit ear. A role for histamine and 5HT in directly
stimulating peripheral nociceptors in acute inflammation seems
to be relatively unimportant because (a) they are at least
1000 times weaker than BK [14] and their concentrations at
the site of inflammation are not likely to reach significant
levels, and (b) in the present study PGE_1 was significantly
more potent in the conscious rat when given 25min after yeast,
ie. at the start of the kinin (second) phase, than when it
was injected at the same time as the yeast.

The third criterion requiring that interference
with the formation, release or action of the mediators should
produce either analgesia or hyperalgesia has been demonstrated
on many occasions including the present studies. In the
anaesthetised cat and dog very small doses of PGE_1, E_2
or $F_{2\alpha}$ potentiated the reflex vasopressor responses to BK
injected into the spleen and reversed the inhibition of
these responses by indomethacin or aspirin. Moreover, in the
conscious rat the hyperalgesia to pressure stimulation induced
by subplantar yeast injections is reversed by nonsteroidal

Table 2 Nociceptor sensitizing actions of prostaglandins in different pain models in animals.

Preparation	Response	PG sensitization; order of potency	Reference
Spleen (anaesth.cat)- close-arterial BK	Reflex vasopressor	$E_1>E_2>F_{2\alpha}>F_{2\beta}>A_1=A_2=0$	This paper
Spleen (anaesth.dog)- close-arterial BK	Reflex vasopressor	$E_1>E_2$ $E_1>E_2>F_{2\alpha}>F_{2\beta}>A_1=A_2=0$	Ferreia et al., 1973 This paper
Knee-joint(anaesth.dog)- BK injection	Reflex vasopressor	$E_1E_2>>F_{2\alpha}=0$	Moncada et al., 1975
Paw (conscious rat)- subplantar yeast	Pressure hyperalgesia	$E_1>E_2>>F_{2\alpha}=F_{2\beta}=A_2=$ $D_2=I_2=0$	This paper
Vasoisolated perfused ear (anaesth.rabbit)- close-arterial BK, 5HT or histamine	Reflex vasodepressor	$E_1>E_2$ [$F_{2\alpha}$ inhibits E_1]	Juan and Lembeck; 1974
Heart (anaesth.dog)- BK superfusion	Reflex vasopressor	$E_1>E_2>F_{2\alpha}>0$	Staszewska-Barczak et al.,1976

antiinflammatory analgesic drugs while nociceptive pressure
thresholds in non-inflamed paws are unaffected[15,17].
The effects of indomethacin and aspirin in these preparations
are most likely due to inhibition of prostaglandin
synthesis[7].

The mechanism by which prostaglandins sensitize
peripheral nociceptors is unknown. Bradykinin is capable of
stimulating the synthesis and release of prostaglandins by
activation of phospholipase A_2 and both BK and PGE_2 are
necessary for nociceptor activation. But the cellular events
involved remain obscure. The order of potency for the nociceptor sensitizing actions of prostaglandins is essentially
the same in different pain models, ie: $PGE_1 > E_2 >> F_{2\alpha} > A_1 = A_2 = D_2 = I_2 = 0$ (Table 2) which suggests that the prostaglandins act
through a specific pharmacological receptor. There are not
many biological systems in which PGE_1 is more potent than
PGE_2. Examples of this are (a) the inhibition of platelet
aggregation [18] but in this model PGI_2 [19] and
PGD_2 [20] are more potent than E_1 while in pain models
they are inactive, and (b) induction of pyresis [21] where
the potency ratios are similar to those for pain and may
therefore be mediated through the same PG receptors. Clearly,
this evidence alone is insufficient but the concept of a
prostaglandin receptor provides a good working hypothesis for
studying the effects of prostanoids on peripheral nociceptors.

ACKNOWLEDGEMENTS

We are grateful to Janine Thomson and M. Skingle for
technical assistance.

REFERENCES

1. Di Rosa, M., Giroud, V.P. and Willoughby, D.A. (1971)
    Studies of the mediators of the acute inflammatory
    response induced in rats in different sites by carrageenin
    and turpentine. J.Path. 104, 15-29.

2. Lim, R.K.S., Guzman, F., Rodgers, D.W., Goto, K., Brown,
    C., Dickerson, G.D. and Engle, R.J. (1964).
    Site of action of narcotic and non-narcotic analgesics
    determined by blocking bradykinin-evoked visceral pain.
    Arch. int. Pharmacodyn. Ther., 152, 25-58.

3. Lim, R.K.S. (1976) Sites of action of narcotic and non-
    narcotic analgesics: mechanism of pain and analgesia.
    Headache, 7, 103-120.

4. Sherrington C.S. (1906). The integrative action of
    the central nervous system Publ. Constable, London.

5. Moncada, S.,Ferreira, S.H., and Vane V.R. (1972)
    Does bradykinin cause pain through prostaglandin
    production. Abstracts of Volunteer Papers.
    V.Int. Congress Pharmacol., San Francisco, 160.

6. Ferreira, S.H., Moncada, S., and Vane J.R. (1971)
    Indomethacin and aspirin abolish prostaglandin-
    release from the spleen. Nature New Biol., 231, 237-239.

7. Vane, J.R. (1971) Inhibition of prostaglandin synthesis
    as a mechanism of action for aspirin-like drugs. Nature
    New Biol., 231, 232-235.

8. Ferreira, S.H. Moncada, S. and Vane, J.R. (1973)
    Prostaglandins and the mechanism of analgesia produced
    by aspirin-like drugs. Br. J. Pharmac. 49, 86-97.

9. Horton, E.W. (1963) Action of prostaglandin E_1 on
    tissues which respond to bradykinin. Nature, 200, 892-3.

10. Crunkhorn, P. and Willis A.L. (1971) Cutaneous reactions
    to intradermal prostaglandins Br.J. Pharmac. 41, 57-64.

11. Ferreira, S.H. (1972) Prostaglandins, aspirin-like drugs
    and analgesia. Nature New Biol. 240, 200-203.

12. Moncada, S., Ferreira, S.H. and Vane, J.R. (1975)
    Inhibition of prostaglandin biosynthesis as the
    mechanism of analgesia of aspirin-like drugs in the dog
    knee-joint. Eur. J. Pharmacol. 31, 250-260.

13.   Staszewska-Barczak, J., Ferreira, S.H. and Vane J.R.,
      (1976) An excitatory nociceptive cardiac reflex elicited
      by bradykinin and potentiated by prostaglandins and
      myocardial ischaemia. Cardiovascular Res., 10, 314-327.

14.   Juan, H., and Lembeck F. (1974) Inhibition of actions of
      E-prostaglandins (PG's) on paravascular pain receptors.
      Naun-Schmeid. Arch. exp. Path. Pharmak. 285, R36.

15.   Winter, C.A. and Flataker, L. (1965) Reaction thresholds
      to pressure in edematous hindpaws of rats and responses
      to analgesic drugs J.Pharm. exp. Ther. 150, 165-171.

16.   Willis, A.L. (1969) Release of histamine, kinin and
      prostaglandin during carageenin-induced inflammation in
      the rat. In: Prostaglandins, Peptides and Amines, Eds.
      Mantegazza, P. and Horton, E.W., 31-38 Acad. Press.
      London/NJ.

17.   Tyers, M.B. Unpublished Observations.

18.   Kloeze, J. (1969). Influence of prostaglandins on
      platelet adhesiveness and platelet aggregation. In:
      Prostaglandins (Proc. 2nd Nobel Symp), Ed. Bergstrom, S.,
      and Samuelsson, B., Interscience, London.

19.   Johnson, R.A., Morton, D.R., Kinner, J.H., Gorman, R.R.,
      McGuire, J.C., Sun, F.F., Whittaker, N., Bunting, S.,
      Salmon, J., Moncada, S., and Vane J.R. (1976). The
      chemical characterisation of prostaglandin X
      (prostacyclin). Prostaglandins 12, 915-928.

20.   Nishizawa, E.E., Miller, W.R., Gorman, R.R., Bundy, G.L.,
      Svensson, J., and Hamberg, M. (1975) Prostaglandin D_2
      as a potential antithrombotic agent. Prostaglandins 9,
      109-121.

21.   Milton, A.S. and Wendlandt, S. (1971) Effects on body
      temperature of prostaglandins of the A, E and F series on
      injection in to the third ventricle of unanaesthetised
      cats and rabbits. J. Physiol (London) 218, 325.

PROSTAGLANDINS AS MEDIATORS OF PYREXIA

W.I. Cranston

There is good evidence that most, if not all, fevers associated with inflammatory or other disease, are caused by the action of endogenous pyrogen (EP), a protein whose monomer has a molecular weight of approximately 14,000 daltons, and which acts on the pre-optic area of the hypothalamus (1-3), and possibly upon another site in the hind-brain (4), setting in train heat conserving and producing mechanisms. Endogenous pyrogen is produced by a variety of cells in the reticulo-endothelial system in response to endotoxin, phagocytosis and other stimuli.

It has been suggested that prostaglandins, probably of the E variety, might play a part in this central action of endogenous pyrogen.

This suggestion rests upon three principal pieces of evidence. Firstly, injection of PGE into the lateral cerebral ventricles causes an almost immediate temperature rise in most, but not all species (5). Secondly, there is an increased concentration of PGE in cerebro-spinal fluid (CSF) during fever induced by the intravenous injection of endotoxin or EP (6). This PGE level is not elevated merely as a consequence of the activation of heat conservation mechanisms, as exposure of animals to a cold environment does not affect the level of PGE in CSF (7). Thirdly, most antipyretic drugs inhibit the synthesis of prostaglandins in brain, by blocking the metabolism of arachidonic acid (AA) to endoperoxides (8). These drugs diminish the febrile response to pyrogens, and prevent the increased concentration of PGE in CSF which normally accompanies fever (6). These three pieces of evidence suggested that PGE might be released as a consequence of the action of EP on the central nervous system, and that PGE might be the final common pathway in the production of fever.

There is, however, some evidence against the direct involvement of PGE in the process. Rabbits treated with the weak antipyretic sodium salicylate, develop a normal fever in response to EP injection, though the rise of PGE concentration in CSF is prevented (9). More convincing evidence against the involvement of PGE in the production of fever was obtained by the use of two antagonists of PGE activity, SC19220 and HR546. These agents, injected into cerebral ventricles, blocked the temperature rise following the intraventricular injection of PGE; neither antagonist had any effect on pyrexia caused by intraventricular injection of EP (10). This makes it unlikely that PGE is itself the mediator of fever, but leaves the possibility that other metabolites of AA could be involved. Laburn et al (11) showed that SC19220 and HR546 did not affect the temperature rise caused by intraventricular injection of AA, though they confirmed that these agents inhibited the temperature rise caused by PGE given by the same route. Indomethacin attenuated the temperature rise following intraventricular AA. This would be compatible with the hypothesis that another metabolite of AA has a function. Investigation of this possibility is difficult, because of the instability of many of the metabolites. The intraventricular injection of prostacyclin does cause temperature elevation, but the dose required is very large - of the order of 100 times larger than the dose of PGE. This may, of course, merely reflect the instability of the compound (12).

It is possible that arachidonic acid metabolites may have nothing to do with the production of fever. Frens et al. (13) found that rats deprived of essential fatty acids, and hence of arachidonic acid, developed a fever identical to that shown by control rats when injected subcutaneously with yeast.

There is some evidence that the pyrexial response to PG, AA and EP may require protein synthesis. Siegert and his colleagues (14) observed that the intravenous injection of cycloheximide (4-5 mg/kg) inhibited the febrile response to intravenous injections of EP. We have confirmed this, and have observed that it also decreases the temperature rise due to intraventricular injections of PGE and AA. Cycloheximide does not appear to interfere with normal central thermoregulation. Whether this effect is due to an action of cycloheximide on protein synthesis, or to some other pharmacological effect, is not yet certain.

REFERENCES

1. Cooper K.E., Cranston, W.I. and Honour, A.J. Observations on the site and mode of action of pyrogens in the rabbit brain. J. Physiol (London) 191:325, (1967).

2. Jackson, D.L. A hypothalamic region responsive to localized injection of pyrogens. J. Neurophysiol. 30:586 (1967).

3. Myers, R.D., Rudy, T.A., and Yaksh, T.L. Fever produced by endotoxin injected into the hypothalamus of the monkey and its antagonism by salicylate. J. Physiol (London) 234: 167, (1974).

4. Rosendorff, D. and Mooney, J.J. Central nervous system sites of action of a purified leukocyte pyrogen. Am. J. Physiol. 220:597, (1971).

5. Milton, A.S. and Wendlant, S. Effects on body temperature of prostaglandins of the A, E, and F series on injection into the third ventricle of unanaesthetised cats and rabbits. J. Physiol (London) 218: 325-336, (1971).

6. Feldberg, W., and Gupta, K.P. Pyrogen fever and prostaglandin-like activity in cerebrospinal fluid. J. Physiol (London) 228: 41-53, (1973).

7. Cranston, W.I., Hellon, R.F. and Mitchell, D. Is Brain Prostaglandin Synthesis Involved in Responses to Cold? J. Physiol (London) 249: 425-434, (1975).

8. Vane, J.R. Inhibition of prostaglandin synthesis as a mechanism of action of aspirin-like drugs. Nature New Biol. 231: 232-235, (1971).

9. Cranston, W.I., Hellon, R.F., and Mitchell, D. A dissociation between fever and prostaglandin concentration in cerebrospinal fluid. J. Physiol (London) 253: 583-592, (1975).

10. Cranston, W.I., Duff, G.W., Hellon, R.F., Mitchell, D. Townsend, Y. Evidence that brain prostaglandin synthesis is not essential in fever. J. Physiol (London) 259: 239-249, (1976).

11. Laburn, H., Mitchell, D. and Rosendorff, C. Effects of prostaglandin antagonism on sodium arachidonate fever in rabbits. J. Physiol (London) 267: 559-570, (1977).

12. Clark, W.G., Lipton, J.M. Hyperthermic Effect of Prostacyclin injected into the Third Cerebral Ventricle of the Cat. Brain Res. Bull. 4: 15-16, (1979).

13.   Frens, J., Van Miert, A.S.J.P.A.M., and Van Duin, C.TH.M.
Prostaglandins are not essential in experimental fever of rats.
Brit. J. Pharmacol. 64: 439, (1978).

14.   Siegert, R., Philipp-Dormston, W.K., Radsak, K. and
Menzel, H.   Mechanism of fever induction in rabbits.   Infect.
immun. 14: 1130-1137, (1976).

MODELS OF ACUTE INFLAMMATION - A COMMENTARY

William Dawson
Lilly Research Centre Limited, Erl Wood Manor,
Windlesham, Surrey GU20 6PH, England

The relevance of models of acute inflammation in
the search for novel anti-inflammatory compounds has long
been a subject for intense discussion. It is assumed that
most chronic inflammatory lesions develop initially as an
acute response to some type of insult to a tissue, be it
viral, bacterial, trauma etc. Subsequently, the character
of the acute reaction changes and the inflammation resolves
or becomes chronic. The real question revolves around the
possible control of the variety of parameters which change
in the acute response by drugs, and whether such control will
modify chronicity.

Using a range of clinically effective anti-
inflammatory compounds, this commentary will attempt to
assess the benefits and disadvantages of acute inflammatory
models. Clinically, the signs and symptoms of acute
inflammation are heat, oedema, erythema and pain. Using
these as the criteria to assess animal models (Table 1),
none of the usual "standard" models reflect all aspects and
it is apparent that measurement of oedema is the most
frequently used parameter. Obviously this is convenient
and objective, although the relevance has been questioned.

Further tests have been developed in an attempt to
characterise the observed functional changes (Table 2). In
particular, pleurisies and implants allow a very reasonable
assessment of cellular and mediator changes, both as the
inflammation develops and also under the influence of drugs.
They can give no guidance on margination and vascular changes.

Table 1   Animal models of acute inflammation

Model	Species	Heat	Oedema	Erythema	Pain
Carrageenin, paw	Rat	-	+	-	-
UV Erythema, skin	Guinea Pig	-	-	+	-
Ear, irritation	Mouse	?	+	+	?
Adjuvant Arthritis (Acute phase), paw	Rat	-	+	-	-
Mild burns, limbs	Rat Mouse	-	+	+	?

Table 2   More definitive animal models of acute inflammation

Model	Species	Heat	Oedema	Erythema	Pain
Pleurisy	Rat Mouse Guinea Pig	-	+	-	-
	plus mediators and cells				
Cheek pouch	Hamster	-	?	-	-
	plus vasculature and perhaps cells				
Blood flow, injured limb	Various	-	?	?	-
	plus vasculature				
Foreign body implant	Rat Mouse Guinea Pig	-	+	-	-
	plus mediators and cells				

In order to study all aspects of inflammation, a range of tests are required. This then requires consideration of spectrum or profile of biological activity, which will be examined in more detail later.

Carrageenin induced paw oedema in the rat is a favourite "acute" model and has often been used as a primary

screen to detect anti-inflammatory activity in novel series
of chemicals. However, the ability of this test to
discriminate between different types of compound, with
different metabolic pathways and half-lives is clearly not
very great (Table 3). Only indomethacin and flurbiprofen
stand out as being rather more potent, but it has proved
difficult in our hands to achieve inhibitions greater than
60-70%. Using the hypothesis that these compounds exert
their activity by inhibiting PG synthetase (Vane 1971) then
either PGs are not totally responsible for acute inflammation
or there must be other mechanisms by which inflammation may
be reduced.

Table 3   Carrageenin paw oedema, effect of drugs

Drug	% Inhibition	
Dose	25 mg/kg* (x2)	50 mg/kg* (x2)
Aspirin	—	20
Ibuprofen	—	28
Phenylbutazone	22	52
Ketoprofen	31	57
Naproxen	24	58
Fenoprofen	32	61
Benoxaprofen	22	52

Indomethacin (0.5 mg/kg x2)	35	
Flurbiprofen (1.0 mg/kg x2)	30	

*Compounds administered orally 3 h and 0.5 h before
 carrageenin.

Paw volumes measured 2.5 h after carrageenin.

n = at least 8.

        The acute phase of adjuvant-induced arthritis in
the rat should, theoretically, be similar to carrageenin
induced inflammation. Relative potencies and dose response
curve slopes are quite different in practice (Table 4)
casting doubt either on common pathogenesis or common mode of
action, a doubt supported by another model of acute inflammation, ultraviolet light induced erythema (Table 5).

Table 4   Adjuvant arthritis in rats, acute phase, effect of
          drugs

Drug/Dose	% Inhibition		
	3 mg/kg	10 mg/kg	33 mg/kg
Phenylbutazone	-	23	29
Naproxen	-	19	32
Ketoprofen	-	39	T
Benoxaprofen	24	27	21
Indomethacin	36	T	-
Flurbiprofen	35	33	-

Compounds administered orally,
each day.

T = toxic

Table 5   Ultraviolet induced erythema in guinea pigs,
          effect of drugs

Drug	ED$_{50}$ (Approx.) mg/kg
Indomethacin	1
Mefenamic acid	13
Phenylbutazone	8
Benoxaprofen	27
Fenoprofen	4

Compounds administered orally 2 h before exposure
to UV light.

Within the chemically diverse area of non steroidal
antiinflammatory compounds, leucocyte migration is a test in
which all compounds are active at concentrations which relate
to their clinical blood levels (Table 6). Interestingly,
however, in an in vivo model in which cellular emigration is
measured, carrageenin induced pleurisy, there is a clear
differentiation between the "standard" compounds assessed.
Fenoprofen and phenylbutazone have no effect (Table 7),
although both have good clinical activity, whilst
benoxaprofen,indomethacin and ketoprofen are active.

Table 6   Effect of Benoxaprofen and other NSAI drugs on the migration of leucocytes _in vitro_ after administration _in vivo_

Compound	Dose mgkg^{-1}	% Reduction in migration	P<
Benoxaprofen	50	37	0.001
Ibuprofen	50	39	0.01
Naproxen	50	44	0.001
Indomethacin	10	11	N.S.
Aspirin	100	44	0.001
Ketoprofen	50	41	0.001
Fenoprofen	50	20	0.05

Cellular emigration induced by intraperitoneal glycogen.
Compounds administered 4 h before glycogen.
Cells harvested 24 h after glycogen.

Table 7   Carrageenin pleurisy in rats

Compound	Dose mgkg^{-1} x 2 p.o.	% Reduction in mononuclears	P<
Benoxaprofen	10	24	N.S.
	25	40	0.001
	50	50	0.001
Indomethacin	2.5	21	N.S.
	5.0	40	0.05
Ketoprofen	50	44	0.001
Fenoprofen	50	No effect	
Phenylbutazone	50	No effect	

Compounds administered 1 h before and 6 h after carrageenin.
Cells harvested 24 h after carrageenin.

There is no correlation between the intrinsic ability of these compounds to inhibit PG synthetase (Table 8) and any of the _in vivo_ models of acute inflammation and it is extremely difficult to correlate either of these activities with clinical efficacy.

Table 8   Inhibition of PG synthetase in vitro

Drug	Bovine Seminal Vesicles IC$_{50}$ μM	Lung IC$_{50}$ μM
Aspirin	30 - 1500	11 - 150
Benoxaprofen	130 - 210	300 - 400
Flurbiprofen	7.0	-
Indomethacin	0.1 - 10	0.1 - 3.5
	2.7 - 3.0	2.6 - 3.7
Phenyl Butazone	88 - 1400	3.0
Naproxen	100 - 370	-
Mefenamic Acid	0.38 - 15	-
Flufenamic Acid	48	0.2

Preincubation time with drug is 3 min
Reaction time is 15 min.

It is clear, therefore, that we lack the correct
test models for correlation, or that the predictive value of
acute inflammatory reactions is not particularly useful.
Prostaglandins undoubtedly play a role in acute inflammation,
but it seems unlikely from this pharmacological data that it
is a central or exclusive role. The complex interactions
between "classical" substances such as the PG's histamine
etc. and cellular products such as peptides, proteins or
phospholipids are obviously fruitful areas of research but it
could well be that better models for such studies will be
found in chronic inflammation.
        Definition of the spectrum of a compound's
biological activity seems to be a necessary prerequisite for
the use of pharmacological agents in studies designed to
increase our knowledge of inflammation, both acute and
chronic. Such a spectrum, as a minimum, should examine
activity on cellular function, relevant biochemical studies
and the vascular responses to the compound in inflammatory
lesions.

Acknowledgements. The considerable help of the anti-inflammatory department of the Lilly Research Centre, and in particular of Dr. S.C.R. Meacock and Miss E.A. Kitchen is gratefully acknowledged.

Reference

Vane, J.R. (1971). Inhibition of prostaglandin synthesis as a mechanism of action for aspirin-like drugs. Nature, New Biology, 231, 232-235.

PROSTAGLANDINS AND THE POLYMORPHONUCLEAR LEUCOCYTE

M.J.H. Smith
Department of Chemical Pathology, King's College Hospital
Medical School, Denmark Hill, London, SE5 8RX.

The migration and accumulation of leucocytes is an
important aspect in the development of inflammatory reactions.
In the earlier stages the predominant cell is the PMN but at
later time periods is succeeded by mononuclear phagocytes (1).
A major difference between the two is that the PMN is a mature
end cell incapable either of proliferation or conversion into
other cell types. It persists in the extravascular spaces and
tissues for a limited time only, a few days at the most.
Nevertheless it could play an important role in both amplifying
and sustaining inflammatory responses. The purpose of the
present article is to review the evidence that it may do so, at
least in part, by interacting with prostaglandin systems. The
information available is largely restricted to intermediates
and products of cyclo-oxygenase pathways from essential fatty
acids (dihomo-γ-linoleic and arachidonic). These include
endoperoxides, prostaglandins and thromboxanes. Attention is
now being increasingly directed to substances formed via
lipoxygenase pathways of the fatty acids necessitating a more
comprehensive and exact nomenclature. However, for con-
venience, the term PGs will be employed to designate prostaglandins and related compounds in this communication.

The general areas of interaction to be considered
comprise the formation of PGs after the release of enzymes by
the PMN, the effects of alterations in cyclic nucleotide
concentrations within the PMN induced by PGs, the biosynthesis
of the PGs by the PMN and the effects of PGs on the behaviour
of the PMN, particularly with respect to its locomotion.

1.   Selective Enzyme Release

The overall aspects of the release of the variety of

enzymes contained with the abundant and characteristic granules
of the PMN, the mechanisms involved and the roles of the
released enzymes and non-enzymatic substances in the production
of inflammation and tissue injury have been discussed in detail
by Davies and Allison (2) and Zurier and Krakauer (3).

There is a large amount of evidence that lysosomal
constituents including acid proteinases, neutral proteinases
and non-enzymatic basic proteins and other PMN enzymes, such as
collagenase, not only act on components of the fluid phase of
exudates to release kinins and activate complement components
but also damage tissues adjacent to the inflammatory site.
This is one interaction of PMNs with PG systems since any
perturbations of cell membranes in the tissue cells will
activate phospholipases. This process will lead to the
production of the precursor fatty acids capable of subsequent
transformation into the cascade of metabolites by the cyclo-
oxygenase and lipoxygenase systems present not only in inflammatory cells, including the PMN, in the exudate itself but also
in a variety of tissue cells at the inflammatory site. Prostaglandin production, being a general property of cells, is a
response of the tissues as a whole and no single cell type is
involved exclusively.

2.   Cyclic nucleotides

The release of lysosomal enzymes from the PMN may be
non-selective such as in acute gout where the phagocytosed
crystals of uric acid are cytolytic. There are also selective
release mechanisms when the PMN either ingests or is exposed to
immune complexes, to cytotaxins (C5a) or to particles coated
with C3b. One factor which may be concerned in the sequence of
events leading to the selective release of lysosomal enzymes by
the PMN is the intracellular concentrations of cyclic nucleotides. Agents which increase cyclic AMP in the PMN reduce
selective release (4) and inhibit directed migration towards
cytotaxins (5). Contrary effects occur when the concentration
of cyclic GMP within the PMN becomes raised. This is another
possible interaction between the PMN and PGs because PGE_1 acts
on suspensions of human peripheral PMNs to elevate their intracellular concentrations of cyclic AMP (6,7), whereas $PGF_{2\alpha}$
increases the levels of cyclic GMP in the PMN (5). There is
evidence (8) in one model of acute inflammation, crystal
induced pleurisy in the rat, that the inflammation only proceeds
normally if the concentration of cyclic AMP in the participatory
leucocytes is lower than in the resting leucocytes. PGE_1 and
other PGs which increase the intracellular concentration of
cyclic AMP in the paw could therefore elicit anti-inflammatory
effects *in vivo*.

In practice such anti-inflammatory actions are produced only by very large pharmacological doses (up to lmg per day) of PGs in various animal models (9). The use of much lower and more realistic amounts (1µg of PGE_1 into an inflammatory exudate) has revealed no anti-inflammatory effects of the prostaglandin until granuloma tissue has become established (10). In the earlier phases of inflammation, when PMNs would be expected to contribute, then the actions of exogenous PGs, PGE_1 as well as PGE_2 and PGI_2, are pro-inflammatory involving the enhancement of blood flow and vasodilatation and the potentiation of plasma exudation (11,12). It does not seem likely that endogenous PGs affect the earlier stages in the development of inflammatory reactions by altering intracellular cyclic nucleotide levels in the PMN.

3.   Biosynthesis of PGs by PMN

A third area of interaction is the biosynthesis of PGs by the PMN. It is not easy to provide direct comparison of the published data since a variety of experimental conditions, assay procedures and stimuli have been employed by different workers. Suspensions of human peripheral PMNs are capable of producing PGs during particle uptake and illustrative data are given in Table 1. In this and succeeding

TABLE 1

PG Formation by Human Peripheral PMNs

Incubation period (min)	Method of assay	Components reported	Amount (ng/10^7 PMNs)		Reference
			resting	stimulated	
120	TLC and RIA	E_1 (E_2: $F_{1\alpha}$: $F_{2\alpha}$)	0.1 0.2	0.5[a] 1.4-2.4[a]	(13)
90	RIA	E_2	1.0	108[b]	(15)
60	RIA, TLC and GC-MS	TXB_2[c]	0.2	0.7[b]	(16)

a - zymosan; b - opsonised zymosan; c - PGs not determined.

tables the experimental results have been recalculated, when necessary, as nanograms produced by a standard number of cells (10^7) and the minor compounds detected are given in brackets.

All the preparations used contained blood platelets varying from a ten-fold excess to a 2.5 per cent contamination but the authors separately assessed the contribution of these platelets in their preparations and concluded that it did not amount to more than 25% of the principal product.

Similar data for elicited (peritoneal) PMNs is contained in Table 2.   There is general agreement that 'resting' cells produce virtually no PGs at incubation periods of up to 2hr but that a variety of stimuli, ranging from addition of arachidonic acid to the ingestion of killed bacteria, cause the biosynthesis of nanogram amounts.   Culture of the cells for 24hr has been reported (23) to cause the production of about 40 to 70ng of E-like material from resting cells with little effect of stimulation ranging from *E.coli* endotoxin to killed *B.pertussis*.   The work of Higgs et al (17) shows that the enzymes necessary for thromboxane synthesis from either PGG_2 or PGH_2 are present in the stimulated elicited rabbit PMN and it has also been demonstrated (18,19) that similar cells produce a monohydroxy and a dihydroxy fatty acid when incubated with arachidonic acid.   These acids are the principal products at short incubation periods (4min) and reflect the activity of lipoxygenase pathways in the PMN.

It has been proposed that the amounts of PGs produced *in vitro* by phagocytosing PMNs appear adequate to account for the concentrations of prostaglandins found in inflammatory exudates of one kind or another (22).   Thus in the exudate formed after 5hr in plastic sponges, impregnated with zymosan, and implanted subdermally in the rat, there are 0.8×10^7 leucocytes and 28ng of PGs per ml (26).   However, it is possible to inhibit the accumulation of leucocytes within the sponge exudate without any corresponding reduction in the content of PGs (27).   In this model, at least, the PGs in the developing exudate must be derived from cells other than the PMN.   A similar experience has been reported by Williams (12) who used a non-allergic model involving the intradermal injection of zymosan in the rabbit and found few PMNs were present on histological examination of the injected sites. Elevated PG levels have been reported by several workers (28-31) in synovial effusions from patients with rheumatoid arthritis.   However, when inflammatory cell populations from either synovial effusions or synovial villi of such patients are cultured *in vitro* and examined for their capacity to produce PGs then the PMN-rich populations from the effusions proved to be poor sources of PGE production compared to the synovial fragments (23).   It was suggested that macrophages were the

TABLE 2

PG Formation by Elicited (Peritoneal) PMNS

Species	Method of assay	Compounds reported	Amount (ng/10^7 PMNs)		Stimulus	Incubation period	Reference
			Resting	Stimulated			
Rabbit	Bioassay	TXA$_2$-like	0	1.5-7.5	Killed bacteria 1h then PGG$_2$ or PGH$_2$	2min	(17)
Rabbit	TLC,GC-MS	Hydroxy eicosa-tetraenoic acids^a	-	-	Arachidonic acid	4min	(18: 19)
Rabbit	Bioassay	E-like	0	0.5-2	Opsonised zymosan	1hr	(21)
Rabbit	GC-MS	TXB$_2$ (F$_{2\alpha}$)	0	1.5-5.5	Opsonised zymosan	1hr	(20: 21)
Rabbit	TLC and bioassay	E1 (E2: F$_{2\alpha}$)	0	4-17	Killed bacteria	2hr	(22)
Rabbit	RIA	E-like	38-72	41-72	Uric acid: Killed Endotoxin: bacteria	24hr	(23)
Rat	RIA	E1 (A1)	0 / 0.4	8 / 22	Ca ionophore / Arachidonic acid	20min / 30min	(24)
Guinea pig	RIA	E-like	3-15	5-36	Uric acid: Killed Endotoxin: bacteria	24hr	(23)

a - These compounds are also formed from arachidonic acid by human peripheral PMNs (25).

major source of local PG formation both in gout and rheumatoid
arthritis (see 32).

4.   Effects of PGs on PMN behaviour
          If it is accepted that PMN suspensions of one to ten
million cells per ml possess the capability to produce nanogram
amounts of PGs then it is pertinent to consider their possible
effects *in vivo*.   The established actions of E-type PGs and of
PGI_2 are pro-inflammatory in that they increase blood flow and
vasodilatation and potentiate the effects of other mediators in
promoting ·increased vascular permeability.   A further possible
pro-inflammatory action of some PGs is as cytotaxins, it having
been suggested that PGE_1 is not only produced by phagocytosing
PMNs but also that it acts as a chemotactic factor for PMNs,
thus playing a controlling role in cellular migration (22).
Most attention has been given to PGE_1 and TXB_2 and the available
data obtained *in vitro* have been summarised in Tables 3-6.
The study of the effects on and mechanisms by which agents of
all kinds affect the locomotion of cells, including PMNs, is
not simply a matter of reporting either a positive or negative
chemotactic response.   Amongst the factors which have to be
both recognised and differentiated in any experimental design
are not only the type of cell, species and methodology but also
the types of movement (random migration, directed migration,
chemokinesis), the effect (chemoattraction, chemotactic modulation, inhibition) and the presence in the sample of other
materials, either of arachidonic acid metabolism or of non-
enzymatic processes, which might be markedly effective at very
low concentrations.   Table 3 lists the reported effects of
PGE_1 on peripheral PMNs.   With the rather obvious proviso that
the concentrations of PGE_1 used are in micrograms rather than
nanograms per ml there is general agreement that freshly
prepared solutions of PGE_1 exert no direct effect on the
migration of peripheral PMNs *in vitro*.   The exception is when
aged, i.e. stored for periods up to months at 4°, solutions of
the PG were employed.   The explanation may well be the presence
of products of non-enzymatic oxidation since it has been
reported (38) that related PGs, such as PGE_2, may be oxidised
in vitro to yield substances which are markedly chemoattractant
for mammalian inflammatory cells.

          The data for elicited PMNs are given in Table 4 where
it is seen that there is consistent evidence that PGE_1 in concentrations of 1µg per ml or less causes a direct chemoattractant effect on rabbit elicited PMNs although not with similar
cells from other species.   However, with the rabbit cells
there are conflicting observations with respect to the modulatory effects of higher concentrations of the prostaglandin on
the movement elicited by conventional stimuli (Table 5).

          The results for thromboxane B_2 are given in Table 6.

TABLE 3

Direct Effects of PGE$_1$ on the Movement of Peripheral PMNs

Species	Concentration (μg/ml)	Effect	Reference
Man	1-100	None	(33)
Man Rabbit	10	None	(34)
Man	1-10	None	(35)
Man Rabbit Rat	1	None	(36)
Rat	1	Increased directed migration (chemoattraction) with aged solutions	(37)

TABLE 4

Direct Effects of PGE$_1$ on the Movement of Elicited PMNs

Species	Concentration (μg/ml)	Effect	Reference
Guinea pig	1	None	(39)
Rat	1	None	(36)
Rabbit	10	None	(34)
Rabbit	4	None	(40)
Rabbit	1	Chemoattraction	(41)
Rabbit	1	Chemoattraction	(42)
Rabbit	1	Chemoattraction	(36)
Rabbit	0.01-1	Chemoattraction	(22)

TABLE 5

Modulatory Effects of PGE$_1$ on the Movement of Elicited Rabbit PMNs

Stimulus	Type	Concentration of PGE$_1$ (μg/ml)	Effect	Reference
Bovine serum albumin	Chemo-kinesin	4	Chemoattraction	(40)
Bacterial Factor	Chemo-attractant	3-1o	Inhibition	(43)

TABLE 6

Direct Effects of TXB$_2$ on the Movement of PMNs

Species	Source	Concentration of TXB$_2$ (μg/ml)	Effect	Reference
Mouse	Elicited	0.5-2	Chemoattraction	(44)
Rat	Elicited	2	Chemoattraction	(45)
Man	Peripheral	0.5-2	Chemoattraction	(45)
Man	Peripheral	1-25	None	(46)

Although microgram per ml concentrations of TXB$_2$ have been reported to exert direct chemoattractant effects on elicited PMNs from rodents there is an apparent conflict of evidence with respect to human peripheral PMNs. One group of workers (45) used biologically prepared material whereas the other (46) employed the synthetic thromboxane. One possible explanation of the discrepant results may be the existence of different mixtures of isomers in the two preparations but an alternative is that during the isolation of the biological material chemoattractant substances were formed by aerobic oxidation processes.

The evidence for PGE$_1$ and TXB$_2$ playing an important role as chemoattractant factors for PMNs *in vivo* is therefore not impressive. If metabolites arising from arachidonic acid, and other fatty acids, by cyclo-oxygenase and lipoxygenase

pathways are concerned in PMN migration in inflammatory
reactions then either HHT (46) or the wealth of hydroxy acids
now being characterised(18,19,25) are potentially more interesting
candidates.

While the migration of PMNs may contribute both to the
exacerbation of acute inflammation and the maintenance of
chronic inflammatory reactions there is little evidence that
interactions with PG systems play either major or specific
roles.   One of the more important facets of PMN involvement in
developing inflammatory responses would appear to be the
selective release of intralysosomal enzymes and the secondary
events which occur as a result.   One of these events may be
the production of prostaglandins and related compounds from
cells and tissues either in a fluid exudate or adjacent to the
inflammatory site.   PGs are, however, only one of a large
group of inflammatory mediators and modulators formed in this
way.

REFERENCES

(1)   R. VAN FURTH, Mononuclear Phagocytes in Inflammation, in
      J.R. VANE and S.H. FERREIRA, Inflammation, (Springer-
      Verlag, Berlin, 1978), p.68-108.

(2)   P. DAVIES and A.C. ALLISON, The Release of Hydrolytic
      Enzymes from Phagocytic and Other Cells Participating in
      Acute and Chronic Inflammation, in: J.R. VANE and S.H.
      FERREIRA, Inflammation, (Springer-Verlag, Berlin, 1978),
      p.267-284.

(3)   R.B. ZURIER and K. KRAKAUER, Lysosomal Enzymes, in: J.R.
      VANE and S.H. FERREIRA, Inflammation, (Springer-Verlag,
      Berlin, 1978), p.285-313.

(4)   G. WEISSMANN, I. GOLDSTEIN and S. HOFFSTEIN, Prosta-
      glandins and the Modulation by Cyclic Nucleotides of
      Lysosomal Enzyme Release, in: B. SAMUELSSON and R.
      PAOLETTE, Advances in Prostaglandin and Thromboxane
      Research, Vol.2 (Raven Press, New York, 1976), p.803-814.

(5)   G.E. HATCH, W.K. NICHOLS and H.R. HILL, Cyclic Nucleotide
      Changes in Human Neutrophils induced by Chemoattractants
      and Chemotactic Modulators, J.Immunol., 119, 450-456
      (1977).

(6)   R.B. ZURIER, G. WEISSMANN, S. HOFFSTEIN, S. KAMMERMAN and
      H.H. TAI, Mechanisms of Enzyme Release from Human Leuco-
      cytes. II.   Effects of cyclic AMP and cyclic GMP.   J.clin.

Invest., 53, 297-309 (1974).

(7) I.R. RIVKIN, J. ROSENBLATT and E.L. BECKER, The Role of
     cyclic AMP in the Chemotactic Responsiveness and Spontan-
     eous Motility of Rabbit Peritoneal Neutrophils, J.Immunol.,
     115, 1126-1134 (1975).

(8) D.A. DEPORTER, C.J. DUNN and D.A. WILLOUGHBY, Cyclic
     Adenosine 3'5'-monophosphate and the Mechanism of Action
     of three common Anti-Inflammatory Drugs, Br.J.Pharmac.,
     65, 163-165 (1979).

(9) M.J.H. SMITH and A.W. FORD-HUTCHINSON, Anti-Inflammatory
     Agents of Animal Origin, in: J.R. VANE and S.H. FERREIRA,
     Anti-Inflammatory Drugs, (Springer-Verlag, Berlin, 1979),
     p.661-697.

(10) I.L. BONTA and M.J. PARNHAM, Time-dependent stimulatory
     and Inhibitory Effects of Prostaglandin E_1 on Exudative
     and Tissue Components of Granulomatous Inflammation in
     Rats.   Br.J.Pharmac., 65, 465-472 (1979).

(11) T.J. WILLIAMS and M.J. PECK, Role of Prostaglandin-
     Mediated Vasodilatation in Inflammation, Nature, Lond.,
     270, 530-532 (1977).

(12) T.J. WILLIAMS, Prostaglandin E_2, Prostaglandin I_2 and the
     Vascular Changes of Inflammation, Br.J.Pharmac., 65, 517-
     524 (1979).

(13) R.B. ZURIER and D.M. SAYADOFF, Release of Prostaglandins
     from Human Polymorphonuclear Leukocytes, Inflammation, 1,
     93-101 (1975).

(14) R.B. ZURIER, Prostaglandin Release from Human Polymorpho-
     nuclear Leukocytes, in: B. SAMUELSSON and R. PAOLETTE,
     Advances in Prostaglandin and Thromboxane Research,
     Vol.2 (Raven Press, New York, 1976), p.815-818.

(15) G. TOLONE, L. BONASERA, M. BRAI and C. TOLONE, Prosta-
     glandin production by Human Polymorphonuclear Leucocytes
     during Phagocytosis *in vitro*, experienta, 33, 961-962
     (1977).

(16) I.M. GOLDSTEIN, C.L. MALMSTEN, H. KINDAHL, H.B. KAPLAN,
     O. RADMARK, B. SAMUELSSON and G. WEISSMANN, Thromboxane
     generation by Human Peripheral Blood Polymorphonuclear
     Leukocytes, J.Exp.Med., 148, 787-792 (1978).

(17) G.A. HIGGS, S. BUNTING, S. MONCADA and J.R. VANE, Poly-
     morphonuclear Leukocytes produce Thromboxane A_2-like

activity during Phagocytosis.   Prostaglandins, <u>12</u>
749-757 (1976).

(<u>18</u>) P. BORGEAT, M. HAMBERG and B. SAMUELSSON, Transformation
of Arachidonic acid and Homo-γ-linoleic Acid by Rabbit
Polymorphonuclear Leukocytes, J. Biol.Chem., <u>251</u>, 7816-
7820 (1976) and <u>252</u>, 8772 (1977).

(<u>19</u>) P. BORGEAT and B. SAMUELSSON, Transformation of Arachidonic
Acid by Rabbit Polymorphonuclear Leukocytes, J.Biol.Chem.,
<u>254</u>, 2643-2646 (1979).

(<u>20</u>) E.M. DAVIDSON, A.W. FORD-HUTCHINSON, M.J.H. SMITH and
J.R. WALKER, The Release of Thromboxane B_2 by Rabbit
Peritoneal Polymorphonuclear Leucocytes, Br. J.Pharmac.,
<u>63</u>, 407P (1978).

(<u>21</u>) E.M. DAVIDSON, M.V. DOIG, A.W. FORD-HUTCHINSON and M.J.H.
SMITH, Prostaglandin and Thromboxane Production by Rabbit
Polymorphonuclear Leucocytes and Rat Macrophages, Advances
in Prostaglandin and Thromboxane Research.   In press.

(<u>22</u>) G.A. HIGGS, E. McCALL and L.J.F. YOULTEN, A Chemotactic
Role for Prostaglandins released from Polymorphonuclear
Leucocytes during Phagocytosis, Br.J.Pharmac., <u>53</u>, 539-
546 (1975).

(<u>23</u>) R.A. STURGE, D.B. YATES, D. GORDON, M. FRANCO, W. PAUL,
A. BRAY and J. MORLEY, Prostaglandin Production in
Arthritis, Ann.Rheum.Dis., <u>37</u>, 315-320 (1978).

(<u>24</u>) B. WENTZELL and R.M. EPAND, Stimulation of the Release of
Prostaglandins from Polymorphonuclear Leukocytes by the
Calcium Ionophore A23187, F.E.B.S. Letters, <u>86</u>, 255-258
(1978).

(<u>25</u>) P. BORGEAT and B. SAMUELSSON, Arachidonic Acid Metabolism
in Polymorphonuclear Leukocytes, Proc.Natl.Acad.Sci.U.S.A.
<u>76</u>, 2148-2152 (1979).

(<u>26</u>) A.W. FORD-HUTCHINSON, J.R. WALKER, N.S. CONNOR and M.J.H.
SMITH, Prostaglandins and leucocyte Migration in Inflammatory Reactions, Agents and Actions, <u>7</u>, 469-472 (1977).

(<u>27</u>) J.R. WALKER, M.J.H. SMITH and A.W. FORD-HUTCHINSON, Anti-
Inflammatory Drugs, Prostaglandins and Leucocyte Migration,
Agents and Actions, <u>6</u>, 602-606 (1976).

(<u>28</u>) L. LEVINE, Antibodies to Pharmacologically Active Molecules:
Specifications and Some Applications of Antiprostaglandins,
Pharmac.Rev., <u>25</u>, 293-307 (1973).

(29) G.A. HIGGS, J.R. VANE, F.D. HART and J.G. WOJTULEWSKI,
      Effects of Anti-Inflammatory Drugs on Prostaglandins in
      Rheumatoid Arthritis, in: H.J. ROBINSON and J.R. VANE,
      Prostaglandin Synthetase Inhibition (Raven Press, New
      York, 1974), p.165-173.

(30) C. PATRONO, S. BOMBARDIERI, O. DIMUNNO, G.P. PASERO,
      F. GRECO, D. GROSSI.BELLINI and G. CIABATTONI, Radio-
      immunoassay Measurements of Prostaglandins $F_{1\alpha}$ and $F_{2\alpha}$
      in Human Synovial Fluids and Superfusates of Human
      Synovial Tissue, in: G.P. LEWIS, The Role of Prosta-
      glandins in Inflammatory (Huber, Vienna, 1975), p.122-137.

(31) D.R. SWINSON, A. BENNETT and E.B.D. HAMILTON, Synovial
      Prostaglandins in Joint Disease, in: G.P. LEWIS, The
      Role of Prostaglandins in Inflammation, (Huber, Vienna,
      1975), p.41-46.

(32) A.W. FORD-HUTCHINSON and M. DOIG, Prostaglandins and
      Macrophages, in: Prostaglandins and Inflammation,(A.W.
      FORD-HUTCHINSON, K.D. RAINSFORD , Birkhäuser Verlag,
      Basel, 1980) p.151.

(33) S.R. TURNER, J.A. CAMPBELL and W.S. LYNN, Polymorphonuclear
      Leukocyte Chemotaxis toward Oxidised Lipid components of
      Cell Membranes, J.exp.Med., 141, 1437-1441 (1975).

(34) J.L. DIAZ-PEREZ, M.E. GOLDYNE and R.K. WINKLEMAN, Prosta-
      glandins and Chemotaxis, J.Invest.Dermatol., 66, 149-152
      (1976).

(35) A. PAZZAGLIA, A. BARKER, A.P. WARIN and M.W. GREAVES,
      Failure of Prostaglandins, Prostaglandin Metabolites and
      Arachidonic Acid to elicit Chemotaxis of Human Polymorpho-
      nuclear Leukocytes, Br.J.Dermatol., 96, 533-536 (1977).
      See also A.R. RABSON, R. ANDERSON, R. LOMNITZER and
      H.J. KOORNHOF, *In vitro* Effects of Prostaglandins on
      Polymorphonuclear Leucocyte Function, South African
      Medical Journal, Supplement, p.44-48 (1974) for report
      of chemoattractant effect of 1-10µg/ml of PGE_1.

(36) J.R. WALKER, M.J.H. SMITH and A.W. FORD-HUTCHINSON,
      Prostaglandins and Leucotaxis, J.Pharm.Pharmac., 28,
      745-747 (1976).

(37) A.W. FORD-HUTCHINSON, M.J.H. SMITH and J.R. WALKER,
      Chemotactic activity of Solutions of Prostaglandin E_1.
      Br.J.Pharmac., 56, 345-346P (1976).

(38) S. SAHU and W.S. LYNN, Lipid Chemotaxins isolated from
     culture filtrates of *E.coli* and from Oxidised Lipids,
     Inflammation, 2, 47-54 (1977).

(39) M.A. BRAY and M.FRANCO, Prostaglandins and Inflammatory Cell
     Movement *in vitrc*, Int.Arch.Allergy Appl.Immunol., 56, 500-
     506 (1978).

(40) G. TILL, E. KOWNATZKI, M. SEITZ and D. GEMSA, Chemokinetic
     and Chemotactic Activity of various Prostaglandins for
     Neutrophil Granulocytes, Clin.Immunol.Immunopathol., 12,
     111-118 (1979).

(41) G. KALEY and R. WEINER, Effect of Prostaglandin E_1 on
     Leucocyte Migration, Nature new Biol., 234, 114-115 (1971).

(42) E.McCALL and F.J.L. YOULTON, Prostaglandin E_1, Synthesis by
     Phagocytosing Rabbit Polymorphonuclear Leucocytes: its
     Role in Chemotaxis.   J.Physiol.Lond., 234, 98-100 (1973).

(43) Reference (7): See also H.R. HILL, R.D. ESTENSEN, P.G.
     QUIE, N.A. HOGAN and N.D. GOLDBERG, Modulation of Human
     Neutrophil Chemotactic Responsiveness, Metabolism, 24,
     447-456, for similar results with peripheral PMNs.

(44) J.R. BOOT, W. DAWSON and E.A. KITCHEN, The Chemotactic
     Activity of Thromboxane B_2, J.Physiol.Lond., 257, 47-48P
     (1976).

(45) E.A. KITCHEN, J.R. BOOT and W. DAWSON, Chemotactic Activity
     of Thromboxane B_2, Prostaglandins and their Metabolites for
     Polymorphonuclear Leucocytes, Prostaglandins, 16, 239-244
     (1978).

(46) E.J. GOETZL and R.R. GORMAN, Chemotactic and Chemokinetic
     Stimulation of Human Eosinophil and Neutrophil Polymorpho-
     nuclear Leukocytes by 12-L-Hydroxy-5,8,10-Heptadecatrienoic
     Acid (HHT), J.Immunol., 120, 526-531 (1978).

NEW VISTAS ON THE ROLE OF PLATELETS IN BRONCHOCONSTRICTIONS.

Michel Chignard, Jean Lefort and Bernardo B. Vargaftig.
Institut Pasteur, 28, rue du Dr. Roux - 75015 PARIS - FRANCE.

I INTRODUCTION

Platelets contain and synthetize a variety of potential inflammatory substances such as histamine, serotonin or prostaglandins.
Other substances such as cationic proteins, elastase or collagenase are also present (Vargaftig, 1977). The release of some
of these substances to the extracellular medium, during platelet
aggregation, is inhibited by non-steroidal anti-inflammatory
drugs. Despite these circumstancial evidences it is generally
believed that platelets do not participate in non-immunological
acute experimental inflammation. This has been supported by results
obtained with the classical model of rat paw oedema induced by
carrageenan, which is not suppressed in thrombocytopenic animals
(Ubatuba et al., 1975). Furthermore, oedema cannot be restored
by platelet administration to leukocyte-depleted animals which
are unresponsive to carrageenan. Finally, oedema is suppressed
by salicylic acid, a drug which fails to block arachidonate-induced platelet aggregation (Vargaftig, 1978).
          Most of the substances, released from platelets during
their aggregation, are potent bronchoconstrictor agents. This is
the case for histamine, serotonin, cyclic endoperoxides, some
primary prostaglandins (Hamberg et al., 1975; Cuthbert, 1973)
and also platelet-activating factor (PAF) (Vargaftig et al.,
1979) which can furthermore be released from platelets themselves (Chignard et al., 1979a). This contribution summarize
recent evidence on interactions of platelets and bronchoconstrictor mechanisms.

II AGGREGATING AGENTS AND BRONCHOCONSTRICTION

Bronchoconstriction was recorded from anesthetized guinea-pigs
by a slight modification of the Konzett-Rössler method (Vargaftig et al., 1971; Lefort and Vargaftig, 1978). Thrombocytopenia was calculated by comparing the platelet counts in whole
blood before and after (10 seconds and 1 minute) intravenous
injection of the drugs.
          All the aggregating agents injected namely arachidonic

acid (AA), collagen, ADP, ATP and PAF induced a transient bronchoconstriction (Table I). A marked drop in the number of circulating platelets was observed concomitantly.

T A B L E   I

COMPARISON BETWEEN BRONCHOCONSTRICTION AND THROMBOCYTOPENIA IN-
DUCED BY SOME AGGREGATING AGENTS.

aggregating agents	doses per kg	bronchoconstriction (cm H_2O)	thrombocytopenia[*] (% of initial count)
ARACHIDONIC ACID	375 µg	15	30
COLLAGEN	75 µg	16	30
ATP	1000 µg	10	60
ADP	100 µg	12	60
PAF	5000 U	8	75

[*] mesured one minute after drug injection, except for ATP and
ADP when it was mesured within 10 seconds.

The thrombocytopenia induced by ATP and by ADP reached its
maximum 10 seconds after injection, whereas for the other drugs
the peak was observed at 1 minute (Table I).
        All the drugs tested, which were selected for their
aggregating properties in vitro, were active in vivo on platelets.
Moreover all induced bronchoconstriction. To what extent can
bronchoconstriction be considered as due to platelet activation?

III PLATELET PARTICIPATION IN BRONCHOCONSTRICTION

Anti-platelet plasma was used to make the guinea-pigs thrombocytopenic. Under such a condition, bronchoconstriction by collagen, ATP, ADP and PAF was completely suppressed, whereas AA-
induced bronchoconstriction was unaffected.
        Bronchoconstriciton by AA can be evoked in isolated
perfused lungs, indicating again that platelets are not required

for the bronchial effect. Nevertheless, the _in vitro_ effect is
not always inhibited by aspirin-like drugs, as would be expected if the only bronchoconstrictor substances present would be
the refered metabolites of AA. A similar situation can be found
for bradykinin, since the _in vivo_ bronchoconstriction is always
blocked by aspirin, whereas the _in vitro_ effect is refractory.
The best available explanation for the discrepancy is that AA
and bradykinin display direct smooth muscle effects, best seen
in vitro and rather irrelevant _in vivo_, where bronchoconstriction is cyclooxygenase-dependent fully.
        It can thus be conclude that all the agents tested,
except AA, induce platelet-dependent bronchoconstriction _in vivo_.

IV PARTICIPATION IN BRONCHOCONSTRICTION OF CYCLOOXYGENASE-
DEPENDENT METABOLITES OF ARACHIDONIC ACID.

Ten minutes after the administration of 5 mg/kg of aspirin I.V.,
the bronchoconstrictor agents were injected. As expected, all
the effects of AA were suppressed. According to the responses,
the other four agents were distributed in two groups. The first
includes ADP and PAF which induced bronchoconstriction unaffected by aspirin and the second includes ATP and collagen, which
induced bronchoconstriction partly and completly blocked by
aspirin respectively (table II). Thrombocytopenia was induced
by all four drugs, and only that due to collagen was affected
by aspirin (table II).
                          T A B L E   II

INTERFERENCE OF ASPIRIN WITH BRONCHOCONSTRICTION AND THROMBOCY-
TOPENIA INDUCED BY SOME AGGREGATING AGENTS

AGGREGATING AGENTS	PERCENT INHIBITION OF	
	bronchoconstriction	thrombocytopenia
ARACHIDONIC ACID	100	100
COLLAGEN	100	20
ATP	70	0
ADP	0	0
PAF	0	0

        In case of ATP and of collagen it appears clearly
that the stimulated platelets released AA-cyclooxygenase
derivatives which are responsible for bronchoconstriction. The
suspected derivatives are prostaglandins F2α, D2, H2 and G2 and
thromboxane A2, which are active either directly (Hamberg et al.,
1975), or via the release from platelets of broncho-active compounds such as serotonin or histamine, this release being inhibited by aspirin (Evans et al., 1968). It is interesting

to note that the accompanying thrombocytopenia was not, or only
partly inhibited by aspirin. This ruled out a direct mechanical
participation of platelet aggregates in bronchoconstriction.
A role for PAF, formed from collagen-stimulated platelets
(Chignard et al., 1979b) and possibly from ATP-stimulated platelets is also ruled out since bronchoconstriction by exogenous
PAF is unaffected by aspirin (Vargaftig et al., 1979). In case
of bronchoconstriction by ADP and by PAF there is no role for
AA-cyclooxygenase derivatives. In case of PAF this is in full
agreement with the fact that it does not induce formation of
prostaglandins and of thromboxanes (Cazenave et al., 1979;
Vargaftig et al., 1979). The release of substances contained in
platelet as an explanation for bronchoconstriction remain an
open possibility, at least in case of PAF. Nevertheless, it has
been demonstrated that serotonin and histamine are not involved
(Vargaftig et al., 1979). Platelet ADP remains as a possible
candidate as cause of PAF-induced bronchoconstriction, but the
bronchial effect of exogenous ADP is platelet dependent and not
direct. The release of as yet unknown smooth muscle stimulating
substances from platelets might thus be anticipated (Vargaftig
et al., 1979).

V INHIBITION OF BRONCHOCONSTRICTION BY PGE1 AND PGI2

PGE1 is a potent bronchodilatator (Rosenthale et al., 1971).
As expected, it prevented all types of bronchoconstriction such
as that induced by collagen or by AA (Vargaftig and Lefort, 1979)
(Table III). Thrombocytopenia induced by AA, and to a lesser
extent that induced by collagen, was also markedly reduced
(Table III). The inhibition of bronchoconstriction is probably

T A B L E   III

INHIBITION BY PGE1 AND BY PGI2 OF BRONCHOCONSTRICTION AND
THROMBOCYTOPENIA INDUCED BY COLLAGEN AND ARACHIDONIC ACID

	PROSTAGLANDIN E1 10 µg/kg % INHIBITION OF		PROSTAGLANDIN I2 1 µg/kg % INHIBITION OF	
	BRONCHO - CONSTRICTION	THROMBO- CYTOPENIA	BRONCHO- CONSTRICTION	THROMBO- CYTOPENIA
COLLAGEN 150 µg/kg	81	56	83	76
ARACHIDONIC ACID 375 µg/kg	65	45	0	70

due to a direct relaxant activity of PGE1 on the bronchial
muscles and not to the inhibition of platelet activation.
Indeed inhibition of thrombocytopenia was less pronounced than
inhibition of bronchoconstriction (Table III). Morevover,
AA-induced bronchonconstriction, which is platelet-independent,
was also inhibited. In contrast PGI2 administered under the
same conditions, i.e. infused for one minute just before the
injection of aggregating agents, did not prevent bronchoconstriction by AA whereas thrombocytopenia was inhibited (Table III).
The same dose of PGI2 (1 µg/kg) inhibited fully bronchoconstriction and thrombocytopenia induced by collagen. Thus PGI2, as
anti-platelet plasma, allows to dissociate platelet-dependent
and platelet independent bronchoconstriction, since it only
suppresses the former. PGI2 was also tested against bronchoconstriction induced by PAF, which was completely inhibited,
as well as the accompanying thrombocytopenia. PGI2 thus prevents
platelet reactivity in vivo, but has no direct effect on the lung
smooth muscle.

CONCLUSION

Even though potential inflammatory mediators are involved in
bronchoconstriction, the latter is not an adequate model for
acute inflammation. In contrast, the association of platelet
and lung studies allow to discriminate sites of action of
potential inhibitors, since the various potential antagonists,
namely anti-histamine, anti-serotonin, anti-inflammatory drugs,
exert precise effects on platelets, on the bronchii, or on both,
depending upon the choosen agonist. Collagen appears as a very
convenient tool, when injected i.v., to study platelet-dependent
bronchoconstriction, whereas AA, as well as bradykinin, allow the
study of platelet-independent bronchoconstriction. The failure
of PGI2 to induce direct bronchodilatation, contrasts with its
effectiveness as antagonist of platelet aggregation, and raises
the important question of the exact role of PGI2 in lungs
(Gryglewski et al., 1978; Moncada et al., 1978), from which it
is secreted. Unless the bronchial reactivity of the human lung
differs markedly from that of the guinea-pig with respect to
PGI2, no role in maintaining the bronchial muscle dilated can be
attributed to it, contrary to PGE2, a recognized bronchodilator
in both humans and guinea-pigs (Cuthbert, 1973). Results in press
(Vargaftig and Lefort, 1979) indicate that anaphylactic bronchoconstriction in the guinea-pig is also unaffected by PGI2, but
also by PGE1. The accompanying thrombocytopenia is also refractory to inhibition by the PGs. Since under those conditions
aggregation in vitro is only obtained in whole blood, but not
in platelet-rich plasma, indicating that its mechanism involves
other cells, it appears that the described model may provide a
new insight into cell activation and bronchial reactivity.
Further work should reveal whether this can be made into a proper
model of allergic asthma.

References

1. CAZENAVE, J.P., BENVENISTE, J. and MUSTARD, J.F., Aggregation of rabbit platelet by platelet-activating factor is independent of the release and the arachidonate pathway and inhibited by membrane-active drugs, Lab. Invest. (in press).

2. CHIGNARD, M., LE COUEDIC, J.P., TENCE, M., VARGAFTIG, B.B. and BENVENISTE, J., The role of platelet-activating factor in platelet aggregation, Nature, 279, 799-800, 1979a.

3. CHIGNARD, M., TENCE, M., LE COUEDIC, J.P., VARGAFTIG, B.B. and BENVENISTE, J., Is platelet-activating factor (PAF) the mediator for the third pathway of platelet aggregation ? Fed. Proc., 38, 1342 abst 5894, 1979b.

4. CUTHBERT, M.F., Prostaglandins and respiratory smooth muscle, in The Prostaglandins : pharmacology and therapeutics advances, by CUTHBERT, M.F., J.B. Lippincott Company, Philadelphia; pp 253-385, 1973.

5. EVANS, G., PACKHAM, M.A., NISHIZAWA, E.E., MUSTARD, J.F. and MURPHY, E.A., The effect of acetylsalicylic acid on platelet function, J. Exp. Med., 128, 877-894, 1968.

6. GARCIA LEME, J.G., BECHARA, G.H. and SANTOS, R.R., A pro-inflammatory factor in lymphocytes. Its role in the development of acute, non-immunological inflammatory reactions, Brit. J. Exp. Pathol., 57, 377-386, 1976.

7. GRYGLEWSKI, R.J., KORBUT, R. and OCETKIEWICZ, A., Generation of prostacyclin by lungs in vivo and its release into the arterial circulation, Nature, 273, 765-767, 1978.

8. HAMBERG, M., HEDQVIST, P., STRANDBERG, K., SVENSSON, J. and SAMUELSSON, B., Prostaglandin endoperoxides. IV. Effects on smooth muscle, Life Sci., 16, 451-462, 1975.

9. LEFORT, J. and VARGAFTIG, B.B., Role of platelets in aspirin-sensitive bronchoconstriction in the guinea-pig; interactions with salicylic acid, Brit. J. Pharmacol., 63, 35-42, 9178.

10. MONCADA, S., KORBUT, R., BUNTING, S. and VANE, J.R., Prostacyclin is a circulating hormone, Nature, 273, 767-768, 1978.

11. ROSENTHALE, M.E., DERVINIS, A. and KASSARICH, J., Bronchodilator activity of prostaglandins E1 and E2, J. Pharmacol. exp. Ther., 178, 541-548, 1971.

12. UBATUBA, F.B., HARVEY, E.A. and FERREIRA, S.H., Are platelets important in inflammation ? Agents and Actions, 5, 31-34, 1975.

13. VARGAFTIG, B.B., Platelets and inflammation, Agents and Actions Suppl. 3, 75-92, 1977.

14. VARGAFTIG, B.B., The inhibition of cyclo-oxygenase of rabbit platelets by aspirin is prevented by salicylic acid and phenanthrolines, Eur. J. Pharmacol., 50, 231-241, 1978.

15. VARGAFTIG, B.B., COIGNET, J.L., de VOS, C.J., GRIJSEN, H. and BONTA, I.L., Mianserin hydrochloride : peripheral and central effects in relation to antagonism against 5-hydroxy-tryptamine and Tryptamine, Eur. J. Pharmacol., 16, 336-346, 1971.

16. VARGAFTIG, B.B. and DAO, N., Release of vasoactive substances from guinea-pig lungs by slow-reacting substance C and arachidonic acid. Its blockade by non-steroid anti-inflammatory agents, Pharmacology, 6, 99-108, 1971.

17. VARGAFTIG, B.B. and LEFORT, J., Interference of prostacyclin and of prostaglandin E1 with anaphylactic shock and with collagen-induced-platelet-dependent and arachidonate-induced platelet-independent bronchoconstriction in the guinea-pig, Prostaglandins (accepted for publication).

18. VARGAFTIG, B.B., LEFORT, J., PRANCAN, A.V., CHIGNARD, M. and BENVENISTE, J. , Platelet lung in vivo interactions : an artifact or a multi-purpose model ?, Haemostasis, (in press).

Summing up: Dr. J.R. Vane

I will start by reinforcing a point Graham Lewis made this morning and that I have made many times.   Inflammation is a multi-mediated response and prostaglandins only contribute to this response alongside the other mediators such as bradykinin, histamine, 5-hydroxytryptamine, lipid peroxides and hydroperoxides. When I first proposed in 1971 that inhibition of prostaglandin biosynthesis could explain the therapeutic and side effects of aspirin-like drugs, PGE_2 was the most likely candidate for the prostaglandin mediation. Now due to many people's work, especially that of our own group and of Samuelsson and colleagues, there are many more potential mediators of the inflammatory response including prostacyclin, thromboxane A_2 and products of the lipoxygenase pathway.   Incidentally, at the International Prostaglandin Conference in Washington in May, E.J. Corey introduced a new term "the eicosanoids", to cover the thromboxanes and products of the lipoxygenase pathway, as well as prostaglandins.   This will be a useful term to embrace all the C20 products of arachidonic acid.

Certainly since the discovery of several other possible mediators we will have to re-assess our earlier evidence that PGE_2 is the main eicosanoid mediator of inflammation.   Since prostacyclin is synthesised by the vessel walls, it could be that this substance contributes to or mediates vasodilatation.

Professor Lewis mentioned the need for specificity of drug effects on the different cyclo-oxygenases.   These are at least three papers showing specificity. Flower and I (1) demonstrated that paracetamol had a more potent effect on cyclo-oxygenase from the brain when compared with that of the spleen. Bhattacherjee and Eakins (2) showed a thousandfold range of activity of indomethacin against cyclo-oxygenases from rabbit spleen (ID50 0.045 μg/ml) and retina (ID50 50 μg/ml). Baenziger et al. (3) have shown that platelet cyclo-oxygenase is more sensitive to aspirin than that of cultured cells from the vessel wall. Certainly we need further explanations for these specificities.   It could be that the second generation of anti-inflammatory compounds, based on the proprionic acids, because they have less gastro-intestinal side effects than the earlier ones are, in fact, demonstrating some of this specificity.

Professor Lewis mentioned the mode of action of glucocorticoids and this was taken further by Dr. Higgs.   The work of Flower (4) has led to the important observation (5) that glucocorticoids initiate synthesis of a peptide which then inhibits phospholipase A_2.   We are now attempting to purify this factor in our laboratories.

Dr. Jones gave us an elegant summary of the pathways involved in the synthesis of the different eicosanoids.   It could be, as Samuelsson suggested in Washington, that there are a whole family of SRSs.   Those of you who are working on SRS and SRS-A should remember that Samuelsson has not claimed that he knows the structure of SRS-A.   He just claims to have found the structure of a SRS and he may well be expected to find several more SRSs as products of the lipoxygenase pathways.

It was interesting that John Westwick was unable to show that the exudation induced by bradykinin could be reduced by indomethacin.   There are many examples (see 6) showing that the effects of bradykinin are partly mediated by prostaglandin release, possibly by prostacyclin release (7) into the circulation.

One of the questions that was not addressed is whether the pro-inflammatory mediator is PGE_2 or prostacyclin, or both.   In this respect one should remember that there are quite a few different observations.   E.A. Higgs et al. (8) showed that prostacyclin is 1/5th as active as PGE_2 in causing oedema in the rat paw, whereas G.A. Higgs et al. (9) showed that prostacyclin is fifty times more active than PGE_2 as a vasodilator in the hamster cheek pouch.   John Westwick tells us that prostacyclin and PGE_2 are equiactive as vasodilators in the rabbit skin. Whether prostaglandin E_2 or prostacyclin are important in a particular situation will depend on the ratio of their activities, how much of each mediator is released and on the duration of release.

There is also the possibility of a diversion of the pathway.   Prostacyclin synthetase is inhibited strongly by lipid peroxides and it could be that a diversion from prostacyclin to prostaglandin E_2 production could have a pro-inflammatory effect, especially taking into account the observation of G.A. Higgs et al. (10) that prostacyclin prevents the margination of leucocytes.

I was glad to hear that Dr. Tyers had confirmed our experiments (see 11) in cats and dogs on the potentiation of bradykinin-induced pain by the various prostaglandins.

Professor Cranston's paper on fever showed that rather unspecific antagonists of prostaglandins did not reduce pyrogen fever.   It appears that those who are looking at fever are at the same stage as people were a few years ago who were looking at prostaglandins in the kidney (see 12).   In the kidney, infusions of arachidonic acid caused renin release and this was abolished by indomethacin. This is very similar to what Professor Cranston said about arachidonic acid-induced fever being reduced by indomethacin.   It was also interesting in the kidney that prostaglandin E_2 did not induce renin release.   We now know that prostacyclin is the mediator of one pathway of renin release and its conversion from arachidonic acid would explain the effects in the kidney.   Perhaps one of the unstable metabolites of arachidonic acid is of importance in mediating pyrogen fever?

Dr. Dawson's experiments showed rather poor effects of aspirin-like drugs on carrageenin oedema and his experimental results are different from those of other workers in this field.   The general experience is that any substance which is well absorbed and also inhibits prostaglandin synthetase has a correlated anti-inflammatory effect.

I think the results reported by Dr. Higgs on the dual inhibition of the different pathways are an important extension of the whole theory on the mode of action of aspirin-like drugs.   The observations described today could bring together inhibition of prostaglandin synthetase and inhibition of cell migration as the main mechanisms of anti-inflammatory activity.   Certainly the results described are just the tip of an iceberg and there will be an explosion of research on lipoxygenase

and inhibitors of this pathway in the next few years.   Already we know that

indomethacin increases cell migration and also increases the release of SRS-A in

anaphylaxis.   We also know that our compound BW755ҫnot only inhibits leucocyte

migration (see Higgs et al., this meeting) but also inhibits the production of SRS-A

in anaphylaxis.

   Professor   Smith   reviewed   very   critically   the   role   of   "PGEs"   and

polymorphonuclear leucocytes in inflammation.   I would like to make a plea that

people should stop talking about "PGEs" as if their activities could be grouped

together. PGE_1 and PGE_2 have quite different activities. For instance, PGE_1 is a

potent inhibitor of platelet aggregation, whereas PGE_2 is not.   In the light of the

discovery of prostacyclin in 1976, we have to re-assess whether PGE_1 has any

relevance to mammalian pathology or physiology.   Where else has its presence

been quite definitively described other than in seminal fluid?.   It could be that in

many experiments in which PGE_1 has been "identified" in inflammatory exudates,

including some of our own, the workers were misled by the fact that there were

background levels of 6-oxo-$PGF_{1\alpha}$ and other eicosanoids of which they were not

then aware.

   It is interesting that Professor Smith mentioned gout in the light of a recent

paper showing that uric acid stimulates prostaglandin production (13).   He also

mentioned PGE_1 as an anti-inflammatory agent and talked about Professor Bonta's

experiments on granulomas.   Once again, I should like to re-affirm that we should

forget about PGE_1 in inflammation but should concentrate in 1979 and onwards on

the role of prostaglandin E_2, prostacyclin and the products of the lipoxygenase

pathway.

1)   Flower, R.J., and Vane, J.R. (1972). Inhibition of prostaglandin synthetase in brain explains the anti-pyretic activity of paracetamol (4-acetamidophenol). Nature (Lond) 240, 410-411.

2)   Bhattacherjee, P. and Eakins, K.E. (1974). Inhibition of the prostaglandin systems in ocular tissue by indomethacin. Br. J. Pharmac. 50, 227-230.

3)   Baenziger, N.L., Dillender, M.J. and Majerus, P.W. (1977). Cultured human skin fibroblasts and arterial cells produce a labile platelet-inhibitory prostaglandin. Biochem. Biophys. Res. Commun. 78, 294-301.

4)   Flower, R.J.   Steroidal anti-inflammatory drugs as inhibitors of phospholipase A_2.   In: Advances in Prostaglandin and Thromboxane Research, eds. C. Galli, G. Galli and G. Porcellati, Academic Press, New York, Vol. 3, pp.105-112, 1978.

5)   Flower, R.J. and Blackwell, G.J. (1979). Anti-inflammatory steroids induce biosynthesis of a phospholipase A_2 inhibitor which prevents prostaglandin generation. Nature (Lond) 278, 456-459.

6)   Vane, J.R. and Ferreira, S.H. (1976). Interactions between bradykinin and prostaglandins. Fogarty Int. Centre Proceedings 27, 255-266.

7)   Moncada, S., Mullane, K.M. and Vane, J.R. (1979). Prostacyclin-release by bradykinin in vivo. Br. J. Pharmac. 66, 96P.

8)   Higgs, E.A., Moncada, S. and Vane, J.R. (1978). Inflammatory effects of prostacyclin (PGI_2) and 6-oxo-$PGF_{1\alpha}$ in the rat paw. Prostaglandins 16, 153-162.

9)   Higgs, G.A., Moncada, S. and Vane, J.R. (1977). Prostacyclin as a potent dilator of arterioles in the hamster cheek pouch. J. Physiol. 275, 30-31P.

10)   Higgs, G.A., Moncada, S. and Vane, J.R. (1978). Prostacyclin (PGI_2) reduces the number of "slow-moving" leukocytes in hamster cheek pouch venules. J. Physiol. 280, 55-56P.

11)   Vane, J.R. (1976). The mode of action of aspirin and similar compounds. J. Allergy & Clin. Immunology 58, 691-712.

12)   Oates, J.A., Whorton, R., Gerber, J., Lazar, J., Branch, R.A. and
      Hollifield, J.W. Prostacyclin and the kidney. In: Prostacyclin, eds. J.R.
      Vane and S. Bergstrom, Raven Press, New York, pp. ??-??, 1979.

13)   Ogino, N., Yamamoto, S., Hayaishi, O. and Tokuyama, T. (1979). Isolation of
      an activator for prostaglandin hydroperoxidase from bovine vesicular gland
      cytosol and its identification as uric acid. Biochem. Biophys. Res. Comm.
      87, 184-191.

Chapter Three

PROSTAGLANDINS AND CHRONIC INFLAMMATION

DISTRIBUTION AND FURTHER STUDIES ON THE ACTIVITY OF PROSTAGLANDIN E IN
CHRONIC GRANULOMATOUS INFLAMMATION

Ivan L. Bonta, Martin J.P. Adolfs and Michael J. Parnham
Dept. of Pharmacology, Erasmus University Rotterdam, P.O.Box 1738,
3000 DR Rotterdam, The Netherlands.

ABSTRACT

        Pre-formed granulomata, induced by cannulated, carrageenin-soaked,
subdermal sponge implants, were used to further analyse the effects of
exogenous PGE and the involvement of endogenous PGE in this model of chronic
inflammatory tissue changes in rats. Experiments with ^{14}C-PGE_2 indicated
that administration of PGE into the sponge creates a kinetic situation likely
to imitate, but superimposed upon, the continuous discharge of endogenous
PGE in the granuloma. The granuloma-reducing, anti-inflammatory effect of
PGE can be mimicked by dibutyryl cyclic-AMP, phosphodiesterase inhibitors
and indomethacin. Most probably these compounds, in common with PGE, exert
their anti-granuloma action through elevation of intracellular cyclic-AMP
(in macrophages and/or fibroblasts). The anti-granuloma action is not
necessarily associated with a reduction in the endogenous PGE-level and vice
versa. The involvement of endogenous PGE in the tissue events of granulomatous inflammation is conjectural as yet.

        INTRODUCTION

        While it is clear that during the acute inflammation prostaglan-
dins (PGs), particularly PGE_2 and/or PGI_2, contribute to vascular, algogenic
and pyrogenic events, the function of PGs in chronic inflammation is the
subject of considerable debate (1,2). Certain aspects of the vascular component of chronic inflammation (e.g. increased blood flow) are promoted by
PGE_1 (3). But the importance of PGE in controlling various tissue aspects -
such as cellular infiltration and function and connective tissue growth - is
unclear, because, depending on the experimental conditions, stimulatory
and inhibitory effects have been reported (1,2). This apparent paradox is
explanable, at least partially, as a time-dependent phenomenon, as shown
with studies on chronic granulomatous inflammation. Thus, PGE_1 promoted
granulomatous tissue growth when administered locally at the time of induction of this type of inflammation, but following administration into pre-
formed granulomata it reduced the mass of the inflamed tissue (4). PGE_2 also

displayed this anti-granuloma action, but equivalent doses of $PGF_{2\alpha}$, PGI_2 and 6-keto-$PGF_{1\alpha}$ failed to exert this effect (5). Granuloma tissue converts exogenously administered arachidonic acid largely to PGE_2, to a smaller extent to $PGF_{2\alpha}$ and even less to PGI_2 (6). It is unkown, as yet, whether the two phenomena, i.e. the sensitivity of granuloma tissue to inhibitory effects of E-type PGs and the property of this tissue to produce mainly PGE_2, are in some way interrelated, although such an association seems likely.

Clinically occurring inflammatory granuloma tissue, for example the pannus of rheumatoid arthritis, is composed of a variety of cell popul- ations, including macrophages, fibroblasts and lymphocytes. But in the carrageenan-impregnated, polyether sponge-induced granuloma of rats - in which the granuloma-reducing anti-inflammatory action of PGE was observed - lymphocytes are not present (7). Macrophages and fibroblasts have thus been proposed as target cell populations of the inhibitory action of PGE in this model (8) and it was subsequently shown that, following treatment of pre- formed granuloma with PGE_1, a significant correlation exists between phago- cytosing macrophages and reduced levels of PGE-like material (PGL) in exu- dates of granulomata (9). In-vitro studies also indicate that PGE_1 induces reversible changes in macrophage morphology, which are associated with in- hibition of phagocytosis (10). In agreement with the anti-granuloma studies in vivo (5), $PGF_{2\alpha}$ failed to inhibit macrophage function in vitro. That fibroblasts in granuloma tissue are probably under the control of PGs, was born out by experiments on rats which were subjected to dietary deprivation of the essential fatty acid precursors of PGs. In such animals, granuloma formation is enhanced and this enhanced tissue growth is associated with increased collagen synthesis (11). While this only indirectly suggests that fibroblasts are targets of PGs, in-vitro studies on cultured fibroblasts provide direct evidence that the growth and/or proliferation of this cell population is inhibited by PGE_1 (12,13).

The mechanism by which PGEs exert their anti-granuloma effect is not exactly known. There are, however, indications that this effect is mediated by stimulation of adenylate cyclase and the subsequent increase in intracellular levels of cyclic-AMP. Pannus formation in adjuvant arthritic rats is inhibited by treatment of these animals with PGE_1, an effect which was enhanced by concomitant administration of an inhibitor of phosphodies- terase (14). The in-vitro inhibitory effect of PGE on fibroblast function is a cyclic-AMP medicated event (12,13) and this is also valid for the in- hibitory action observed on macrophages (10,15). A cyclic-AMP mediated mechanism has been proposed as the most likely basis for the in-vivo anti- granuloma action of PGE (8). Subsequent to this proposal, it was found that the granuloma-reducing effect of PGE_1 is abolished by SQ-22536, an adenylate cyclase antagonist (16). Furthermore, the anti-granuloma action of PGE is mimicked by inhibitors of phosphodiesterase and to some extent by dibutyryl cyclic-AMP (17).

The findings enumerated above have been observed with exogenously administered PGE. Accordingly, the anti-granuloma action of PGE is a pharma- cological effect. Nevertheless, there are also observations which are con- sistent with the view that endogenous PGE, released during granulomatous in- flammation, modulates the process through actions on cell populations from which the granuloma tissue is composed (2,8,9,11,17). These observations, however, only provided indirect evidence and therefore did not allow clear

conclusions to be drawn. The experiments to be discussed in the present
paper have been designed to further elucidate the effect of PGE on pre-
formed granulomata and to examine further a possible involvement of endogenous PGs in chronic granulomatous inflammation.

METHODS

        Granulomatous inflammation was induced in male Wistar rats (170-
200g) by subdermally implanted, carrageenan-soaked polyether sponges with
indwelling cannulae, as described elsewhere (18), each rat receiving 2
implants. The cannulae were exteriorised at the back of the neck and per-
mitted the injection of substances to be made into the sponge implants at
any chosen time during the different phases of granuloma development. The
size of the implanted sponges was half of that described in the original
method. Effects of the injected compounds were assessed 8 days after implantation in terms of granuloma dry weight, according to the procedure
reported previously (18). Exudates from 8 day-old granulomata were obtained
by a centrifugation technique also described elsewhere (19). The concentration of PGE-like material (PGL) in exudates was bioassayed, after extraction, by a laminar flow superfusion method (20,21). In one experiment, PGs
were extracted not only from the exudates, but also from the sponges and
bioassayed as PGL. In an attempt to obtain an indication of the distribution
of PGE after treatment of a pre-formed granuloma, ^{14}C-PGE$_2$ (1 µCi/10 µg,
Radiochemical Centre, Amersham) was injected through the cannula into one of
the sponges, 4 days after implantation into a rat (Fig.1).

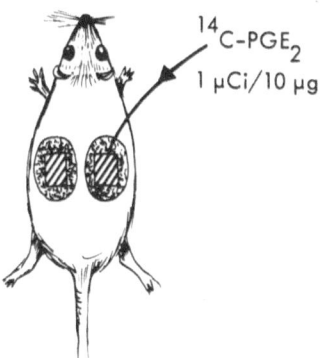

^{14}C-PGE$_2$

1 µCi/10 µg

5 hours after administration
scintillation counts in:
 • injected sponge + granuloma
 • uninjected   "   "
 • expired CO_2
 • urine
 • various organs

Figure 1.   Schematic representation of experiment to examine the fate
             of PGE$_2$ injected into sponge implant.

The animal was attached to a device for trapping $^{14}CO_2$ in the expired air
(22) and samples were collected for counting by liquid scintillation at 15
minute intervals over a period of 5 hours, during which urine was also collected. At the end of the 5 hours, the rat was sacrificed, the injected and
the contralateral sponges removed, together with the granuloma-tissue and
various organs and all tissues and urine were subjected to counting for
radioactivity.

Except for the experiment with $^{14}C-PGE_2$, drugs were administered
via the cannulae in all other experiments 4-7 days after sponge implantation
at the daily doses specified in the table and the figures. All the drugs
were dissolved in saline, an equivalent volume of which was injected into
the concomitantly treated control rats.

RESULTS AND DISCUSSION

Distribution of PGE

Despite the large number of experiments in which the highly reproducible anti-granuloma effect of PGE has been established (4,5,9,16,17),
no information has hitherto been obtained concerning the fate of the PGE
after it is injected into the sponge implant at a time when a well formed
granuloma has grown around the implant. Data on the physical holding capacity of the sponge implant (18) do not indicate the fate of the PGE given to
a sponge with an established granuloma, which anyway has a high degree of
vascularization and in which PGE administration causes a further increase in
blood flow (3). Thus, the administered PGE is likely to be taken up into
the circulation and metabolized or transported to other organs. The question
we sought to answer was to what extent this occurs. Five hours after the
administration of $^{14}C-PGE_2$, the treated sponge contained the largest portion
of the injected label, the surrounding granuloma contained little radioactivity, while considerable amounts were detectable in the expired air and
apparently very little was excreted via the urine (Fig. 2).
The presence of $^{14}CO_2$ in the expired air is almost certainly the consequence
of β-oxidation of the hydro-carbon chain of the injected PGE_2. Furthermore,
the 5 hour value shown in Fig.2 is well below the peak value for this parameter, which was observed 1h 30 min after the $^{14}C-PGE_2$ administration (Fig.3).
While the portion of the label in the treated sponge was only determined 5
hours after $^{14}C-PGE_2$ administration (Fig.2), it is likely, from the time-
course of the expired $^{14}C-CO_2$, that the label in the sponge must have been
present in a much higher proportion at an earlier period after the injection.
The verification of this assumption is the subject of current experiments to
be reported elsewhere. These experiments have also been designed to show
whether the proportional distribution of the label between the sponge and
the surrounding granuloma tissue displays time-dependent variations.

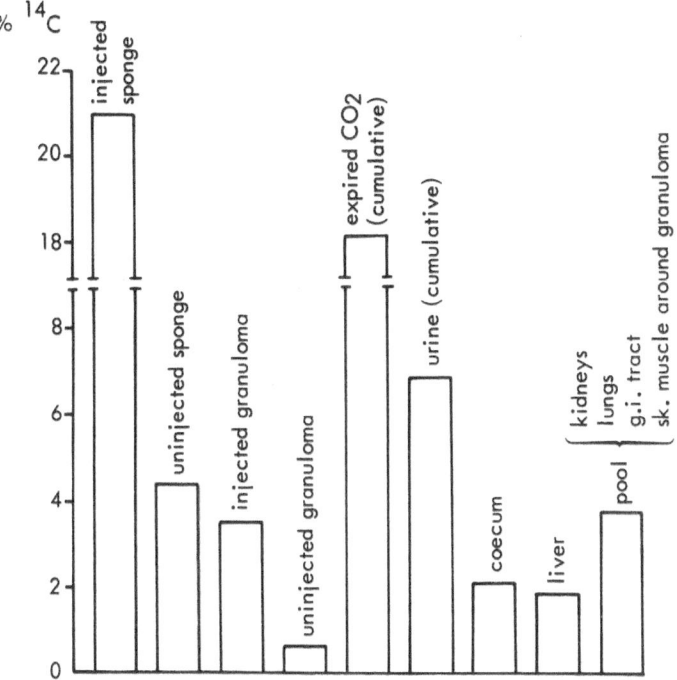

Figure 2.   Distribution of ^{14}C-label 5 hours after injection of ^{14}C-PGE$_2$
             into a 4-day old sponge implant.

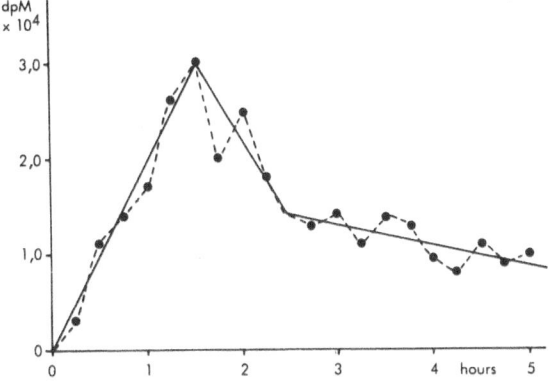

Figure 3.   Expired ^{14}C-CO$_2$ after administration of ^{14}C-PGE$_2$ (1 µCi/10 µg)
             into a 4-day old sponge implant. Each point indicates a
             separate measurement of an air sample collected over a 15 min
             period.

Granuloma tissue has a low capacity to metabolize PGs by 15-
dehydrogenase (discussed in ref.1 and 6), but other metabolic pathways are
conceivable. Obviously, the presence of the ^{14}C-label does not indicate
per se the presence of the biologically active PGE_2. Bearing these reservations in mind, the present tentative measurements nevertheless indicate
that, provided PGE is administered at a time when granuloma tissue is already present, the sponge implant serves as a depot from which the injected
PG is slowly released into the surrounding inflamed tissue. In this way,
the experimental design of administering PGE into the sponge implant with an
already established granuloma, appears to be a reasonable, though somewhat
exaggerated, model of the natural situation. In the latter, a permanent
release of PGE_2 occurs from the infiltrating macrophages and fibroblasts (2).
That the situation described here is an exaggeration is obvious, since the
exogenous PGE is superimposed upon the outflow of the endogenous substance.
This circumstance is one of the complicating factors which make it difficult
to conclude whether the pharmacological, anti-granuloma effect is analogous
to a conceivably similar, but as yet unproven, function of endogenous PGE
(see discussion of ref.9).

Mimickry of anti-granuloma effect of PGE

The proposal that the anti-granuloma effect of PGE is mediated
through elevation of intracellular cyclic-AMP levels (8), prompted us to
examine whether a reduction of granuloma tissue can be achieved by increasing
cyclic-AMP levels with other substances. It was subsequently shown that some
inhibitors of phosphodiesterase induced an anti-granuloma effect which was of
a similar order of magnitude as that produced by PGE_1 (17). With dibutyryl
cyclic-AMP (db-cAMP), however, the effect, though qualitatively similar,
failed to reach significance. Nevertheless, despite local administration to
the inflamed site, db-cAMP seemed to stimulate the adrenal cortex (unpublished data), which probably turned on a systemic negative feed-back on the
pituitary-adrenal axis. Whether this might have, to some extent, mitigated
the anti-granuloma effect of db-cAMP is uncertain, but the possibility was
not inconceivable. An attempt was thus made to determine whether treatment
of rats with metyrapone - a recognized procedure to achieve chemical ablation
of the adrenal cortex - would provide improved conditions to demonstrate a
granuloma-reducing effect of db-cAMP. In agreement with previous results
(17), db-cAMP did slightly reduce the granuloma weight in normal rats, but
in metyrapone-treated animals the effect was much more pronounced, to the
extent of becoming highly significant (Table 1).

The above postulated mechanism, by which metyrapone treatment may
have facilitated the anti-granuloma effect of db-cAMP, still remains to be
proven. But what is more important is that, in any case, a means was found
to disclose this inhibitory effect. Thus, the concept that the granuloma-
reducing, anti-inflammatory effect of PGE is mediated by elevation of cyclic-
AMP is supported by the findings that (i) the effect is counteracted by a
blocker of adenylate cyclase (16) and (ii) it is simulated by inhibitors of
phosphodiesterase (17) and by db-cAMP, as shown here. In addition, it appears that adrenaline or isoprenaline administration to pre-formed granulomata is also an effective way to achieve an anti-granuloma effect (to be
published). This suggests that the β-adrenergic catalytic subunit of adenylate cyclase, is also a sensitive site to produce a granuloma-reducing, anti-

Table 1.   Anti-granuloma effect of dibutyryl cyclic-AMP

Rats	Dry granuloma weight (mg)	
	Saline	db-cAMP (mg)
Normal	520 + 40	420 + 30
Metyrapone treated	510 + 40	360 + 40***

Metyrapone treatment consisted of s.c. administration
of 40 mg/kg on days 4 and 5, followed by 20 mg/kg on
days 6 and 7. Db-cAMP was administered according to the
time schedule described in the Methods section. Values
are means + SEM from 5 rats (10 granulomata) per treatment group. Significance (saline v. db-cAMP) was determined by the one-tailed Mann Whitney U test. *** P<0.01.

inflammatory effect.   This set of data seem to justify the cautious conclusion that an in-vivo anti-granuloma action can be exerted by a variety of
agents, provided that they elevate cyclic-AMP levels in the cell populations
involved (e.g. macrophages, fibroblasts).   In this sense, PGE can be considered as a physiological model compound, which serves as a prototype for
a mode of action.which may turn out to be a pharmacological blue print in
the search for new drugs in the treatment of the tissue component of chronic
inflammation.   This proposal has already been advocated previously (2,8,16,
17).

Anti-granuloma action and levels of endogenous PGL

        While some earlier data indicated that a granuloma-reducing effect
is correlated with a reduction of PGL levels in 8-day old granulomatous
exudate (17), contradictory results have been also reported (9) and a further
study of this matter was necessary.   We have now measured the two parameters
in parallel, following the administration of PGE$_1$ and RA-233 [2,6 bis(di-
ethanolamino)-4-piperidino-pyrimido (4,5d) pyrimidine] .   The latter compound is a potent inhibitor of phosphodiesterase (23) and has been shown to
display an anti-granuloma action (17).   In the present experiment, the reducing effect on granuloma weight was confirmed for both PGE$_1$ and RA-233
(in the presence of metyrapone), but while with PGE$_1$ this effect was not associated with any change in endogenous PGL-concentration, RA-233 caused a
drastic fall in PGL levels (Fig.4).   Furthermore, the combined administration
of the two compounds exerted the same effect on granuloma weight and PGL
concentration as did RA-233 when given alone.

        It is obvious that granuloma tissue weight and endogenous PGL
production were influenced independently of each other and it appears that
reduction of PGL-discharge is not the mechanism through which the inhibitor
of phosphodiesterase mimicked the anti-granuloma action of PGE$_1$.   Previous
studies have shown that 24h after the last injection, exogenous PGE$_1$ does
not interfere with PGL determination (9,17).   The chronic anti-inflammatory
effect of PGE$_1$ in adjuvant arthritic rats was shown to be enhanced by concomitant administration of a phosphodiesterase inhibitor (14).   Such a potent-

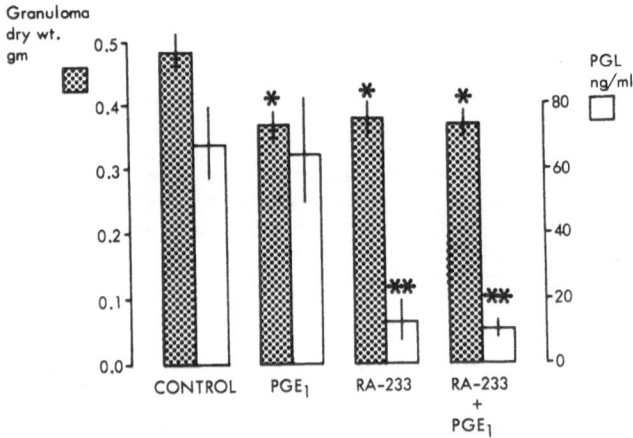

Figure 4.   Effects of PGE$_1$ (1 µg) and RA-233 (20 µg) on granuloma dry
             weight and PGL concentration, which was measured in the pooled
             extracts from sponges and exudates. All rats received metyra-
             pone treatment at the dose shown in the legend to Table 1.
             The compounds were administered according to the time schedule
             described in the Methods section. Values are means $\pm$ SEM from
             5 rats (10 granulomata and 5 PGL values) per treatment group.
             Significance (control v. drug) was determined by one tailed
             Mann Whitney U test. * $P<0.05$, ** $P<0.025$.

iation is not observable in the carrageenan-soaked sponge-induced granuloma
model.   Infiltrating lymphocytes are not involved in the pathogenesis of the
latter model (7), whereas lymphocytes represent a cell population, which
plays a pivotal role in adjuvant arthritis.   It is, thus, possible that the
involvement of lymphocytes is a factor which determined whether PGE$_1$ and an
inhibitor of phosphodiesterase potentiate the chronic anti-inflammatory effect one of the other. However, this explanation does not exclude other
possibilities, which have been discussed elsewhere (2,17).

        Parallel measurements of granuloma weight and endogenous PGL levels
were also performed after administration of indomethacin to pre-formed
granulomata (Fig.5). At the dose employed, indomethacin exerted an anti-
granuloma action, which was associated with a very marked reduction of endogenous levels of PGL. Administration of PGE$_2$ (2 µg), together with indomethacin, counteracted the anti-granuloma action without appreciably influenc-
ing the drop in the concentration of endogenous PGL. The indomethacin-
induced changes in both parameters were abolished with a higher dose of PGE$_2$.

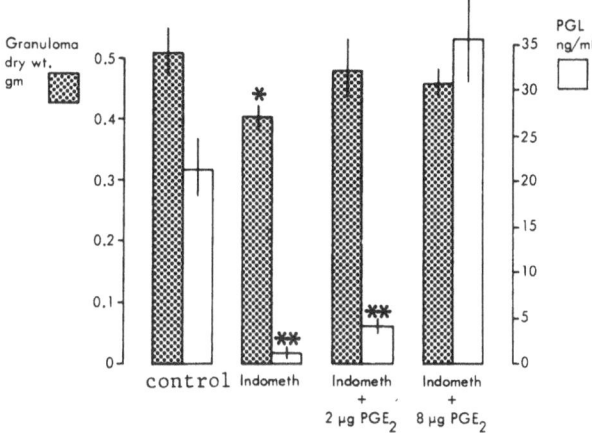

Figure 5.   Effects of indomethacine (200 µg) alone and in combination
             with PGE$_2$ on granuloma dry weight and PGL concentration in
             8-day old granulomatous exudate. The compounds were admin-
             istered according to the time schedule described in the
             Methods section. Values are means ± SEM from 5 rats (10
             granulomata and 5 PGL measurements) per treatment group.
             Significance control v. drug) was determined by one tailed
             Mann Whitney U test. * P<0.05, *** P<0.01.

The granuloma-reducing anti-inflammatory effect of indomethacin was more
pronounced when a higher dose was administered (data not shown), but such a
dose was markedly toxic, i.e. causing the death of 2 out of the 5 treated
rats. It thus appears that a non-toxic dose of indomethacin produces only
a moderate inhibitory effect on the tissue component of chronic inflammation.
This corroborates similar observations made by others (24,25). The present
experiment shows that the anti-granuloma action of indomethacin is of the
same order of magnitude as that usually observed with either PGE or an inhibitor of phosphodiesterase (see Fig. 4 and ref. 4,5,9,16,17). In addition,
it should be emphasized that the anti-granuloma actions of PGE and inhibitors
of phosphodiesterase display a plateau (unpublished observations), similar
to that seen with a non-toxic dose of indomethacin. Recent studies by others
have indicated that indomethacin elevates intracellular cyclic-AMP levels
in vitro (26). It is therefore not inconceivable that this mechanism,
rather than inhibition of cyclo-oxygenase, explains the anti-granuloma action
of indomethacin. It is possible that a cyclic-AMP mediated anti-granuloma
action can only achieve a circumscribed limit, but further studies (including
direct measurement of cyclic-AMP metabolism in granuloma tissue or in cell
populations from such tissue) are needed to disclose this. With regard to
the lack of parallellism between the reduction of granuloma weight and endogenous PGL levels, the results demonstrated in Fig. 4 and 5 are in close
agreement with each other. The administration of PGE in combination with
indomethacin did not reduce the granuloma weight as it does when given alone,

but rather reversed the reduction. This paradox is almost certainly associated with the fact that the exogenous PGE is superimposed upon the discharge of the endogenous PG. Accordingly, the pharmacological effect of
PGE may depend on the eventual level of PGE at the inflamed site. This complicating factor has been discussed earlier in this paper. Finally, the
two sets of experiments (Fig. 4 and 5) taken together do not seem to provide
much support for the idea that endogenous PGL might play a very important
role in the proliferative component of granulomatous inflammation.

CLOSING REMARKS

        The present study is a continuation of a series of papers in which
the granuloma-reducing anti-inflammatory effect of PGE was investigated.
In two of these papers, the phenomenon is described (4,5), while in others
(9,16,17) attempts were made to explain the mechanism through which this
effect is exerted. In the present work, more evidence in favour of a cylic-
AMP mediated mechanism has been presented. It is almost certain that macrophages and fibroblasts are the cell populations which form the target of
this inhibition and current studies are aimed at disclosing this. Although
the anti-granuloma action of PGE is exerted at a dose which is close to
pathophysiological concentrations, it should once more be emphasized that it
is a pharmacological effect. While it cannot be said that this pharmacological effect is a mimickry of a similar function of endogenous PGE, the
available evidence does not allow a conclusion to be drawn one way or the
other.

Acknowledgements

        Peter C. Bragt, M.Sc. kindly provided assistance with the device
to collect and measure $^{14}CO_2$ in the expired air. Thanks are due to the
pharmaceutical house, Dr. Karl Thomae GmbH (Biberach an der Riss), for a
gift of RA-233. Financial support was provided by the Nederlandse Vereniging
tot Rheumatiekbestrijding (Dutch Association to Combat Rheumatism).

REFERENCES

(1)   I.L. BONTA and M.J. PARNHAM, Prostaglandins and Chronic Inflammation,
       Biochem.Pharmac. 27, 1611-1623 (1978).
(2)   M.J. PARNHAM and I.L. BONTA, Prostaglandins and Granuloma Formation
       in vivo. In: Connective Tissue Changes in Rheumatoid Arthritis and the
       Use of Penicillamine (Eds. I.L. Bonta and A. Cats). Agents and Actions
       Suppl. (In press, 1979).
(3)   M.J. PARNHAM, L.D. DE LEVE and P.R. SAXENA, Development of Enhanced
       Blood Flow Responses to Prostaglandin E_1 in carrageenan-Induced
       Granulation Tissue, Agents and Actions (In press, 1979).

(4)   I.L. BONTA and M.J. PARNHAM, Time-Dependent Stimulatory and Inhibitory
        Effects of Prostaglandin E1 on Exudative and Tissue Components of
        Granulomatous Inflammation in Rats, Br.J.Pharmac. 65, 465-472 (1979).
(5)   M.J. PARNHAM, I.L. BONTA and M.J.P. ADOLFS, Distinction Between Pros-
        taglandin E2 and Prostacyclin as Inhibitors of Granulomatous Inflamma-
        tion, J.Pharm.Pharmac. (In press, 1979).
(6)   P.C. BRAGT and I.L. BONTA, In Vivo Metabolism of $1-^{14}C$ Arachidonic
        Acid During Different Phases of Granuloma Development in the Rat,
        Biochem.Pharmac. 28, 1581-1586 (1979).
(7)   P.C. BRAGT, I.L. BONTA and M.J.P. ADOLFS, Cannulated Teflon Chamber
        Implant in the Rat: A New Model for Continuous Studies on Granulomatous
        Inflammation, J.Pharmacol.Meths. (In press, 1979).
(8)   I.L. BONTA and M.J. PARNHAM, Chronic Inflammatory Conditions and
        Mechanisms by Which They May Be Modulated by Prostaglandin-E, Europ.J.
        Rheum.Inflam. 2, 97-103 (1979).
(9)   M.J. PARNHAM, I.L. BONTA and M.J.P. ADOLFS, Modulation of Granulomatous
        Inflammation by Prostaglandin E. Involvement of Mononuclear Cells.
        In: Arachidonic Acid Metabolism in Inflammation and Thrombosis. (Eds.
        K. Brune and M. Baggiolini) Agents and Actions Suppl. (In Press, 1979).
(10)   R.L. OROPEZA-RENDON, V. SPETH, G. HILLER, K. WEBER and H. FISCHER,
        Prostaglandin E1 reversibly induces morphological charges in macropha-
        ges and inhibits phagocytosis, Exp.Cell Res. 119, 365-371 (1979).
(11)   M.J. PARNHAM, S. SHOSHAN, I.L. BONTA and S. NEIMAN-WOLLNER, Increased
        Collagen Metabolism in Granulomata Induced in Rats Deficient in Endo-
        genous Prostaglandin Precursors, Prostaglandins 14, 709-714 (1977).
(12)   H.D. PETERS, B.A. PESKAR and P.S. SCHONHOFER, Influence of Prostaglan-
        dins on Connective Tissue Cell Growth and Function, Naunyn-Schmiede-
        berg's Arch.Pharmacol. 297, S89-S93 (1977).
(13)   P.S. SCHONHOFER, W. RUCKER, A. DEMBINSKA-KIEC, H.D. PETERS, B.A. PESKAR
        and K. von FIGURA, Prostaglandins and fibroblast functions in vitro.
        In: Connective Tissue Changes in Rheumatoid Arthritis and the Use of
        Penicillamine. (Eds. I.L. Bonta and A. Cats). Agents and Actions Suppl.
        (In press, 1979).
(14)   I.L. BONTA, M.J. PARNHAM and L. VAN VLIET, Combination of theophylline
        and prostaglandin E1 as inhibitors of the adjuvant-induced arthritis
        syndrome of rats, Ann.Rheum.Dis. 37, 212-217 (1978).
(15)   M.J. WEIDEMANN, B.A. PESKAR, K. WROGEMANN, E.Th. RIETSCHEL, H. STADINGER
        and H. FISCHER, Prostaglandin and Thromboxane Synthesis in a Pure
        Macrophage Population and the Inhibition, by E-type Prostaglandins,
        of Chemiluminescence, FEBS Letts. 89, 136-140 (1978).
(16)   M.J. PARNHAM, M.J.P. ADOLFS and I.L. BONTA, Alteration of Granuloma
        Formation by PGE1: Effects of an Adenylate Cyclase Inhibitor and
        Splenectomy. In: P. Ramwell, B. Samuelsson and R. Paoletti, Advances
        in Prostaglandin and Thromboxane Research, Vols.6&7 (Raven Press, New
        York, 1979) in press.
(17)   I.L. BONTA, M.J. PARNHAM and M.J.P. ADOLFS, Mimickry of Anti-Granuloma
        Effect of Prostaglandin E by Dibutyryl Cyclic-AMP and Some Phospho-
        diesterase Inhibitors. In: Arachidonic Acid Metabolism in Inflammation
        and Thrombosis (Eds. K. Brune and M. Baggiolini) Agents and Actions
        Suppl. (In press, 1979).
(18)   I.L. BONTA, M.J.P. ADOLFS and M.J. PARNHAM, Cannulated Sponge Implants
        in Rats for the Study of Time-Dependent Pharmacological Influences on
        Inflammatory Granulomata, J.Pharmacol.Meths. 2, 1-11 (1979).

Bonta et al.   132

(19) G.A. HIGGS, E.A. HARVEY, S.H. FERREIRA and J.R. VANE, The Effects of
      Anti-Inflammatory Drugs on the Production of Prostaglandins in vivo,
      In: B. Samuelsson and R. Paoletti, Advances in Prostaglandin and
      Thromboxane Research, Vol1 (Raven Press, New York, 1976) pp.105-110.
(20) S.H. FERREIRA and F. DE SOUZA COSTA, A Laminar Flow Superfusion Tech-
      nique with Much Increased Sensitivity for the Detection of Smooth
      Muscle-Stimulating Substances, Eur.J.Pharmacol. 39, 379-381 (1976).
(21) H. BULT, M.J. PARNHAM and I.L. BONTA, Bioassay by Cascade Superfusion
      Using a Highly Sensitive Laminar Flow Technique, J.Pharm.Pharmac. 29,
      369-370 (1977).
(22) B.H. LAUTERBURG and J. BIRCHER, Expiration Measurement of Maximal
      Aminopyrine Demethylation In Vivo: Effect of Phenobarbital, Partial
      Hepatectomy, Portacaval Shunt and Bile Duct Ligation in the Rat,
      J.Pharmac.Exp.Ther. 196, 501-509 (1976).
(23) D.C.B. MILLS and D.E. MACFARLANE, Stimulation of Human Platelet
      Adenylate Cyclase by Prostaglandin D_2, Thromb.Res. 5, 401-412 (1974).
(24) M. FUKUHARA and S. TSURUFUJI, The Effect of Locally Injected Anti-
      Inflammatory Drugs on the Carrageenin Granuloma in Rats, Biochem.
      Pharmac. 18, 475-484 (1969).
(25) E. KULONEN and M. POTILA, Effect of the Administration of Antirheumatic
      Drugs on Experimental Granuloma in Rat, Biochem.Pharmac. 24, 219-225
      (1975).
(26) D.A. DEPORTER, C.J. DUNN and D.A. WILLOUGHBY, Cyclic Adenosine 3'5'-
      monophosphate and the Mechanism of Action of Three Common Anti-Inflam-
      matory Drugs, Br.J.Pharmac. 65, 163-165 (1979).

PROSTAGLANDINS AND CHRONIC INFLAMMATION

J. Morley, Clinical Pharmacology Unit, Cardio-Thoracic Institute,
Fulham Road, London SW3 6HP.

Diseases in which chronic inflammation is a dominant feature
are commonly of unknown aetiology, so that treatment is necessarily symptomatic. Anti-inflammatory drugs in current use
have been selected on this basis and much effort continues to be
expended in clinical trials designed to compare novel with
established compounds. It is natural therefore, that attempts
should be made to circumvent this cumbersome process by defining
the mode of action of anti-inflammatory drugs in mechanistic
terms. The discovery that synthesis of prostaglandins (PGs) was
inhibited by therapeutic concentrations of a group of the anti-
inflammatory drugs, the non-steroidal anti-inflammatory drugs
(NSAIDs), led to the proposition that this was the mechanism
responsible for the anti-inflammatory effects of these drugs.(1).
It is timely to make an appraisal of this hypothesis.

Firstly, the PGs should themselves be examined as potential
mediators of chronic inflammation as this is a necessary pre-
condition of the hypothesis. Despite considerable biological
potency on many tissues, PGs were not actively considered as
inflammatory mediators prior to this hypothesis. This was
because of their failure to adequately fill the role of a
mediator of acute inflammtion(2) and emphasis of their attributes
as inflammatory mediators has largely been a consequence of the
circular argument that if NSAIDs inhibit PG synthesis then PGs
must be inflammatory mediators. The capacity of E-type PGs to
produce vasodilatation was well established prior to 1971; their
capacity to cause increased vascular permeability and pain
rested on a less certain foundation until it was shown that, in
these two test systems, they act in conjunction with other
mediators as potentiating agents (3,4). Thus PGs, and in
particular PGE_2, possess the necessary properties to evoke dolor,
rubor, turgor and calor (i.e. the classical features of acute inflammation). That much said, the question arises as to whether
they have the capacity to evoke features of chronic inflammation
additional to these actions. They certainly have some further
properties of relevance to chronic inflammation such as an effect
on bone resorption (5) and collagen synthesis (6). However, they

have proved somewhat ineffectual in tests relating to the
accumulation and activation of mononuclear and other cells,
which would seem an essential property of a mediator of chronic
inflammation. One might fairly conclude that the properties of
PGs are more appropriate to primary mediator of acute rather
than chronic inflammation.

     The second and direct question is to consider to what
extent the efficacy of NSAIDs is related to (and can be predicted from) their potency as inhibitors of PG synthesis.
Inevitably this is difficult since it raises the question of
relative efficacy of drugs in chronic inflammation, a topic
which could only be resolved by enormous multi-centre, multi-
drug trials. Nonetheless, it is possible to make pertinent
observations. Carageenin oedema is a widely used test of anti-
inflammatory efficacy in animals. Consequently it is possible
to compare the efficacy of drugs as inhibitors of this
inflammatory process (in terms of ED_{50} values) with the efficacy
of the same drugs as inhibitors of PG synthesis (Figure 1).

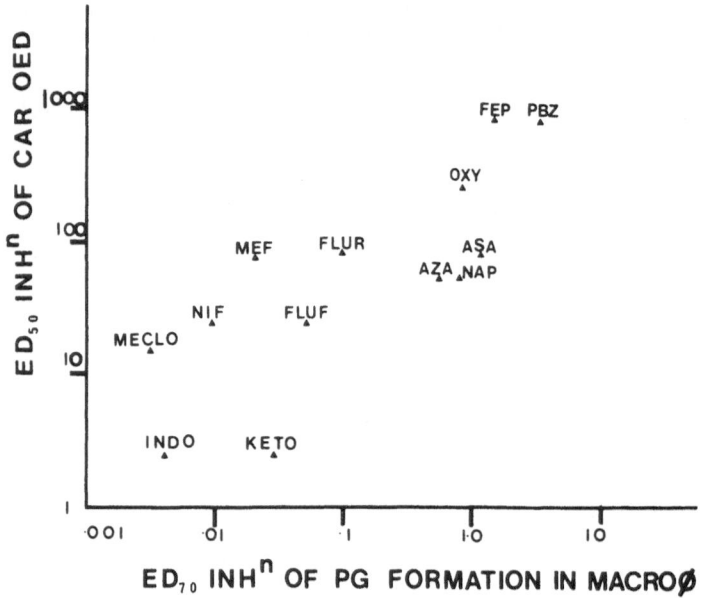

FIGURE 1.   Correlation of efficacy as an inhibitor of
carageenin oedema with efficacy as an inhibitor of prostaglandin
formation.

This exercise is not especially objective since much latitude
exists in selection of ED_{50} in both tests.   For the present
purposes it seemed that data derived from tissue culture studies
(7) was more akin to the in vivo situation than studies on
enzyme preparations.   The selection of ED_{50} values for carrageenan oedema employed a standard text (8), though it is
acknowledged that data derived from less diverse studies is to
be preferred.   Notwithstanding these difficulties, it is
possible to demonstrate that broadly there is a correlation
between capacity to inhibit PG synthesis and efficacy as inhibitors of carrageenin oedema.   From this, it follows that one
can predict anti-inflammatory efficacy (in carrageenin oedema)
from PG synthesis inhibition data.   The question that naturally
follows is whether PG synthesis inhibition is also predictive of
anti-inflammatory efficacy in man.

Comparative studies of NSAIDs tend to be restricted com-
parisons of few drugs at few doses so that there is no ready way
of collecting data on man equivalent to ED_{50} values in carrageenin oedema.   However, individual companies do recommend
doses or dose ranges for their products on the basis of their
collective experience.   It is suggested that these doses would
at least include equieffective doses and hence be suitable for
plotting against potency in PG synthesis inhibition (Figure 2).

It can be reasoned that if NSAIDs act in chronic inflammation by virtue of PG synthesis inhibition, then the product of
the potency and the equieffective dose should be a constant.
Rather than being a constant, the product of potency and dose in
man showed a greater than 500 fold variation.   Interestingly,
there was correlation between this product and the potency in PG
synthesis inhibition there is a need for proportionately greater
doses of drug.   This could be interpreted as indicating not
only that there are other bases of anti-inflammatory actions in
these drugs but also that the efficacy as specific cyclo-.
oxygenase inhibitors is actually counter productive in terms of
over-all anti-inflammatory action, i.e. that PGs may exert some
significant anti-inflammatory action.

The anti-inflammatory action of PGs has been noted for some
time (9).   Actions of such massive doses of PGs are in themselves of only academic interest, however, the case for their
participation as anti-inflammatory agents is strengthened by
observation of an anti-inflammatory/immunosuppressive effect of
precursor fatty acids (10) and by the use of dietary depletion
of the precursors, which moreover both exacerbates the severity
of experimental allergic encephalitis (11) and permits demonstration of an anti-inflammatory effect of PGs at low dosage
(12).

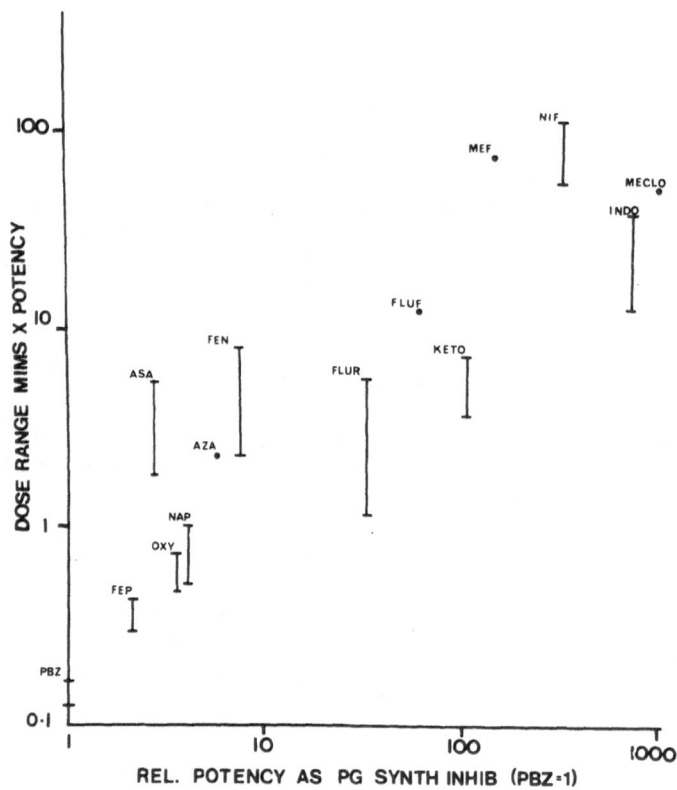

FIGURE 2. Plot of the product of potency and dose range (Monthly Index of Medical Specialities) with potency as inhibitor of PG synthesis. Should anti-inflammatory dose be determined simply by potency as an inhibitor of PG synthesis, the potency dose product would be constant.

The question naturally arises as to how PGs might exert such an effect at the cellular level. The potency of PGs as inhibitors of cell activation in a variety of cell types (13) certainly gives them the theoretical capacity for such an effect. However, the participation of this type of process in chronic inflammation must be linked to identification of a particular cell type as a primary agency of the pathogenesis of chronic inflammation and the demonstration that such a cell is susceptible to inhibition by PG application. Although not defi-

nitively established, it is increasingly evident that the
pathogenesis of rheumatoid arthritis (R.A.) involves lymphocytes and in particular small lymphocytes as primary agents.
This view is based on: (a) The circumstantial evidence of
immunological disfunction in R.A. i.e. rheumatoid factor production; (b) The histological evidence of lymphocytic infiltration in synovial lesions; (c) the efficacy of thoracic duct
drainage in cases of severe R.A.; and perhaps the most compel-
ling observations; (d) The intense inflammatory response evoked
by injection of thoracic duct cells into a quiescent joint (14).
To this could be added the considerable potential of lymphocytes
to effect tissue damage (e.g. in graft rejection) which can be
attributed to cytotoxic action of activated lymphocytes or to
secreted products of lymphocyte activation (lymphokines) which
have a variety of properties appropriate to a mediator of
chronic inflammation (15). It is not unreasonable therefore,
to postulate lymphokine secretion as a central agency in R.A.
and to examine PG actions on this type of cell.

     It has been know for some time that E type PGs would
inhibit lymphocyte activation in vitro (16). Subsequently this
was demonstrated in guinea-pigs in which both antigen activation
and concommitant lymphokine secretion were shown to be inhibited by PGE_1 and E_2 in a dose related manner (17,18). The
effective concentration range was 10-1,000ng/ml which is somewhat higher than levels reported in inflammatory effusions in
man, though it should be noted that the sensitivity of human
cells to PGE_2 inhibition using corresponding test systems is
somewhat greater (19). This type of data provides evidence
of a mechanism whereby PGE may exert a potential anti-inflammatory role. However, it does not in itself establish this
mechanism as physiological.

     An indication that PGE inhibition of lymphokine secretion
might be a physiological, as opposed to a pharmacological,
phenomenon was provided when PG-like materials were sought in
lymphokine preparations. Although at this time (1974) much
emphasis was given to neutrophils as a source of E-Type PGs, it
soon became apparent that macrophages were much more likely
sources of PGs in inflammatory effusions (17), a view confirmed
by a study of human synovial material from patients with
active R.A. (20). The levels of PG achieved over 24 hour incubation of guinea-pig macrophages (usually in the range of
10-100 ng/ml) were sufficient to suggest that active
inhibition of lymphocytes could be achieved and this inference
was confirmed by the action of low concentrations of indomethacin, which enhance lymphokine secretion. Thus the elements of
a negative feed-back system exist in that lymphocytes can be
inhibited by PGE_2, macrophages produce PGE_2 and the juxtaposi-
tion of these cells, together with the concentration of PGs in
bulk solution and the effect of indomethacin indicate that
this regulatory effect can be achieved in vitro. It should be

noted that a more dynamic analysis is needed for a more searching test of this hypothesis.

However, greater interest perhaps attaches to the possible operation of this system in man. A number of groups have demonstrated this type of phenomenon using human cells, particularly Goodwin and co-workers (21) who have suggested that the source of PGE_2 in peripheral blood cells is a large adherent lymphocyte acting as a suppressor T-cell. They have sought the involvement of this system in a variety of diseases in which immunodeficiency is evident and present strong evidence that it underlies anergy in a series of patients with Hodgkins disease (22). These patients showed impaired lymphocyte stimulation which could be fully reversed by indomethacin whilst in vitro leucocyte culture yeilded a high level of PGE_2, whose production was indomethacin sensitive. The logical extension of this is to determine whether indomethacin treatment in vivo increase skin reactions of delayed hypersensitivity and though this is not reported in these patients, it is a phenomenon that can occur in some forms of immunodeficiency (23).

The foregoing is sufficient evidence to merit the consideration of anti-inflammatory (immunosuppressive) effects of PGs in chronic inflammation. It seems likely that these phenomena are not restricted to the test systems described and could contribute in other parts of the inflammatory response (e.g. cell accumulation mechanisms) in which detailed experimental analysis remains to be undertaken. A quite serious question must now be posed, namely do NSAIDs exacerbate the inflammatory responses? This of course, depends on the extent to which lymphocytes (or other cells) in chronic inflammation are susceptible to PGE_2 inhibition. It has been proposed (24) and evidence presented (25) that loss of reactivity to PGE_2 is a feature of lymphocytes which act as primary agencies of chronic inflammation. The evidence on this remains inconclusive and tests on cell populations such as thoracic duct cells would be definitive in this matter. If on the other hand these cells are susceptible to PGE_2 inhibition then it can be predicted that NSAIDs would enhance secretion of pathogenic material. Some evidence in support of this prediction is provided in synovial explant studies in which PGE_2 and collagenase secretion in response to lymphokine stimulation were studied. On a number of occasions it has been observed that whilst PGE_2 formation was strongly inhibited, collagenase production was enhanced (26). Against this others (27) have reported to PGE formation is an obligatory prerequisite for in vitro lymphokine activation of guinea-pig macrophages to secrete collagenase.

An attempt has been made to present evidence that in chronic inflammation PGE_2 is involved not solely as a mediator but also as a regulator of, amongst other cells, T-lymphocytes. The

relevance of this hypothetical relationship to human disease
depends upon the extent to which it can be shown to operate
in vivo, since the nature of in vitro conditions may be quite
critical in the demonstration of this anti-inflammatory effect
of PGs. The work on unsaturated fatty acid deficient animals
as well as certain limited clinical data suggest that such
immunosuppressive/anti-inflammatory effects of PGs are operative
in human disease and that this phenomenon should be considered
in the design and selection of anti-inflammatory drugs. As a
concept it is not without precedent for a closely analogous
situation is evident in asthma. In asthmatic subjects NSAIDs
are generally inert however, in a small proportion (aspirin-
sensitive patients) aspirin and other NSAIDs produce a severe
bronchospasm. Recent challenge studies (28) have clearly
established that sensitivity to provoking drugs is related to
their capacity to inhibit cyclo-oxygenase. Although initially
explained in terms of loss of PGE_2 inhibitory action of mast
cell degranulation or smooth muscle tone, it now seems more
probably associated with diversion of arachidonic acid metabolism
to lipoxygenase pathways and concomitant   increased production
of SRS-A. Of greater importance to the present argument is
that in this disease NSAIDs can exacerbate the disease process,
albeit in only a subpopulation of patients. The detection of
aspirin sensitivity is aided by the dramatic life threatening
response to the drug, by the objective measurements of response
afforded by lung function tests and by the absence of any
beneficial (bronchodilator) effects of aspirin (except on very
rare occasions). It does not seem too great a burden on the
imagination to consider that a parallel position may exist in
rheumatoid arthritis especially since it has been proposed that
the mast cell is a T-cell derivative (29).   It is to be hoped
that rheumatologists might explore this possibility for further
investigation of this hypothesis can best be undertaken in an
appropriate clinical environment.

(1)   J.R. VANE and S.H. FERREIRA. New aspects of the mode of
      action of non-steroidal anti-inflammatory drugs. Ann.
      Rev. Pharmacol.,14 57-73 (1974).

(2)   E.W.HORTON. Action of prostaglandin E_1 on humans which
      respond to bradykinin. Nature, 200, 892 (1963).

(3)   S.H. FERREIRA. Prostaglandins, aspirin-like drugs and
      analgesia. Nature New Biol. 240, 200-203 (1972).

(4)   T.J. WILLIAMS and J. MORLEY. Prostaglandins as potentiators
      of increased vascular permeability in inflammation.
      Nature, 246, 215-217 (1973).

(5)   M. HARRIS, M.V. JENKINS, A. BENNETT and M.R. WILLIS
      Prostaglandin production and bone resorption by dental
      cysts. Nature, 245, 213-215 (1973).

(6) H.D. PETERS, B.A. PESKAR and P.S. SCHONHOFER. Influence
     of prostaglandins on connective tissue cell growth and
     function. Archives of Pharmacology, 297, 89-93 (1977).

(7) M.A. BRAY and D. GORDON. Prostaglandin production by
     macrophages and the effect of anti-inflammatory drugs.
     Brit. J. Pharmacol. 63, 636-642 (1978)

(8) R.S. SCHERRER and M.W. WHITEHOUSE. "Anti-inflammatory
     agents". Academic Press: New York (1974).

(9) R.L. ASPINALL and P.S. CAMMARATA. Effect of prostaglandin
     E_2 on adjuvant arthritis. Nature, 224, 1320-1321 (1969)

(10) J. MERTIN and D. HUGHES. Specific inhibitory action of
     polyunsaturated fatty acids on lymphocyte transformation
     induced by PHA and PPD. Int. Arch. Allergy Appl. Immunol.,
     48, 203-210 (1975).

(11) J. CLAUSEN and J. MØLLER. Allergic encephalomyelitis in-
     duced by brain antigen after deficiency in polyunsaturated
     fatty acids during myelination. Is multiple sclerosis a
     nutrative disorder? Acta Neurol. Scand., 43, 375-388
     (1967).

(12) I.L. BONTA and M.J PARNHAM. Time-dependant stimulatory
     and inhibitory effects of prostaglandin E_1 on exudative
     and tissue components of granulomatous inflammation in
     rats. Br. J. Pharmacol., 65, 465-472 (1979).

(13) S. BERGSTROM. Prostaglandins: Members of new hormonal
     system. Science, 157, 382-391 (1967).

(14) C.M. PEARSON. Should one stimulate or suppress the immune
     response in the rheumatic diseases? In "Infection and
     Immunology in the Rheumatic diseases" (ed. D.C. Dumonde),
     Blackwell: Oxford pp 535-539 (1976).

(15) J. MORLEY. Lymphokines in "Inflammation: Handbook of Exp.
     Pharmacol." (eds. J.R. Vane and S.H. Ferreira) Springer-
     Verlag: New York, 50, (1), 314-342 (1978).

(16) J.W. SMITH, A.L. STEINER and C.W. PARKER. Human lymphocyte
     metabolism. Effects of cyclic and non-cyclic nucleotides,
     on stimulation by phytohaemagglutinin. J. Clin. Invest.
     50, 442-448 (1971b).

(17) M.A. BRAY, D. GORDON and J. MORLEY. Role of prostaglandins
     in reactions of cellular immunity. Br. J. Pharmacol.,
     52, 453P (1974).

(18) D. GORDON, M.A. BRAY and J. MORLEY. Control of lymphokine
     secretion by prostaglandins. Nature, 262, 401-402 (1976).

(19) J. MORLEY, P.J. KIRBY, J.R. PONSFORD and W.I. McDONALD.
     Leucocyte reactivity to prostaglandins in multiple sclerosis.
     In "Immunopathology of nervous diseases" Proceedings of
     Merarimi Foundation Symposium (1977) (ed. P.A. Miescher),
     in press.

(20) R.A. STURGE, D.B. YATES, D. GORDON, M. FRANCO, W. PAUL,
     M.A. BRAY and J. MORLEY. Prostaglandin production in
     arthritides. Ann. Rheum. Dis., 37, 315-320 (1978).

(21) J.S. GOODWIN, A.D. BANKHURST and R.P. MESSNER. Suppression
     of human T-cell mitogenesis by prostaglandin. Existence
     of a prostaglandin producing suppressor cell. J. Exp. Med.,
     146, 1719-1734 (1977).

(22) J.S. GOODWIN, R.P. MESSNER, A.D. BANKHURST, G.T. PEAKE
     J.H. SAIKI and R.C. WILLIAMS. Prostaglandin producing
     suppressor cells in Hodgkin's disease. N. Eng. J. Med.,
     297, 963-968 (1978).

(23) J.S. GOODWIN, A.D. BANKHURST, S.A. MURPHY, D.S. SELINGER,
     R.P. MESSNER and R.C. WILLIAMS, Jr. Partial reversal of
     the cellular immune defect in common variable immuno-
     deficiency with indomethacin. J. Clin. Lab. Immunol., 1,
     197-199 (1978).

(24) J. MORLEY. Prostaglandins and lymphokines in arthritis.
     Prostaglandins, 8, 315-326 (1974).

(25) P.J. KIRBY, J. MORLEY, J.R. PONSFORD and W.I. McDONALD.
     Defective PGE reactivity in leucocytes of multiple sclerosis
     patients. Prostaglandins, 11, 621-630 (1976).

(26) J-M. DAYER, S.R. GOLDRING and S.M. KRANE. Connective
     tissue resorption and rheumatoid arthritis: synovial cell
     cultures as a model. In "Proc. Mech. of localised bone
     loss" (eds. J.E. Horton, T.M. Tarpley and W.F. Davis) pp
     305-308. Inf. Ret. Inc.: U.S.A. (1978).

(27) L.M. WAHL, C.E. OLSEN, S.M. WAHL, A.C. SANDBERG and S.N.
     MERGENHAGEN. Prostaglandin regulated macrophage collagenase.
     In "Proc. Mech. of localised bone loss" (eds. J.E. Horton,
     T.M. Tarpley and W.F. Davis) pp. 181-190. Inf. Ret. Inc.:
     U.S.A. (1978).

(28) A.SZCZEKLIK, R.J. GRYGLEWSKI, G. CYERNIAWSKA-MYSIK.
     Relationship of inhibition of prostaglandin biosynthesis by
     analgesics to asthma attacks in aspirin-sensitive patients.
     Br. Med. J., 1, 67-69 (1975).

(29) F.M. BURNET. Possible identification of mast cells as
     specialised post-mitotic cells. Medical Hypotheses, 1,
     3-5 (1975).

MACROPHAGES RESPONDING TO INFLAMMATORY STIMULI SYNTHESISE INCREASED AMOUNTS OF PROSTAGLANDINS

P. Davies,* R. J. Bonney,* J. L. Humes[+] & F. A. Kuehl Jr.[+]

Dept. Immunology[*] and Biochemistry[+]
Merck Institute for Therapeutic Research
P. O. Box 200
Rahway, New Jersey 07065   U.S.A.

1. INTRODUCTION

The concept of the macrophage as a secretory cell has emerged following many experimental observations showing that cells of the mononuclear phagocyte lineage release soluble substances into their pericellular environment (for reviews see Ref 1,2). Such observations have been made in tissue culture systems where the static environment allows the accumulation of released substances or their breakdown products. It has been much more difficult to demonstrate such phenomena in in vivo situations since released products are disseminated into the extracellular environment and are also subject to inhibition or inactivation by endogenous substances.

The molecular mechanisms underlying the interaction of inflammatory stimuli with membrane components of phagocytic cells have not been elucidated. It is therefore not possible to provide an explanation of the biochemical events that lead to the synthesis and secretion of various mediators by these cells. For this reason our discussion of the synthesis of arachidonic acid oxygenation products will be confined to (a) establishment of the source of substrate arachidonic acid and (b) the description of conditions under which its oxygenation is stimulated by inflammatory stimuli.

2.   SOURCES OF ARACHIDONIC ACID IN MONONUCLEAR PHAGOCYTES

Studies on both human and rabbit alveolar macrophages indicate that phospholipids comprise up to eighty per cent of the total lipids of these cells, neutral lipids and cholesterol esters accounting for the bulk of the remaining lipid (3). The major phospholipid is phosphatidylcholine, with phosphatidylethanolamine, sphingomyelin, phosphatidylserine and phosphatidylinositol being other phosphatides present.   The highest proportion of arachidonic acid is contained in phosphatidylethanolamine, phosphatidylserine and phosphatidylinositol, ranging from eleven to eighteeen per cent of the total fatty acid content. Phosphatidylcholine contains three per cent arachidonic acid (3).

Earlier studies on human peripheral blood monocytes (4) showed that arachidonic acid constituted twenty per cent of the total fatty acid content of cellular phospholipids. Mason et al (5) reported that arachidonic acid constituted nineteen per cent of the total fatty acid content of cellular phospholipid of rabbit alveolar macrophages.

Free arachidonic acid is esterfied at a rapid rate by mononuclear phagocytes. Cultures of resident peritoneal macrophages from specific pathogen free mice or elicited in mice by intraperitoneal injection of one of a variety of inflammatory stimuli incorporate ^{3}H-arachidonic acid rapidly into cellular phospholipids (6). Resident cell populations incorporate forty to sixty per cent of label within four hours while cells from stimulated animals incorporated approximately sixty per cent of label in four hours (6). Analysis of cellular phospholipids showed that the bulk of the label was incorporated into phosphatidylcholine and phosphatidyl-ethanolamine in both cell populations although significantly greater proportions of the label was found in triacylglycerol in the stimulated populations. Very little label remained unesterfied in thoroughly washed cultures (6).

3. SYNTHESIS OF ARACHIDONIC ACID OXYGENATION PRODUCTS BY MONONUCLEAR PHAGOCYTES

There are now many studies showing that mononuclear phagocytes secrete certain arachidonic acid oxygenation products. We have reviewed these studies elsewhere (2, 7,8), and a summary of this is given in Table 1. Prostaglandin E$_2$ appears to be a major product of most mononuclear phagocyte populations studied. Some populations also synthesize prostaglandin I$_2$, thromboxane A$_2$, prostaglandin F$_{2\alpha}$ and products of the lipoxygenase pathway (9). The basal rate of production of oxygenation products by cultured mouse peritoneal macrophages is not great as measured by production of labeled products from cells prelabeled with ^{3}H-arachidonic acid or by radioimmunoassay for prostaglandin E (6). However as shown below this basal rate can be greatly increased by inflammatory stimuli.

4. THE STIMULATION OF THE SYNTHESIS OF ARACHIDONIC ACID OXYGENATION PRODUCTS BY MOUSE PERITONEAL MACROPHAGES RESPONDING TO STIMULI OF ACUTE AND CHRONIC INFLAMMATION.

In view of the well established function of the macrophage as a secretory cell and indications by other workers (10, 11) that mononuclear phagocytes secrete oxygenation products of arachidonic acid, we investigated the fate of ^{3}H-arachidonic acid preincorporated into mouse peritoneal macrophages upon exposure of these cells to model inflammatory stimuli. In our initial experiments we chose zymosan since this particulate stimulus has been shown to be a potent inducer of chronic inflammation in a number of situations (12,13). Zymosan added to cultures of unstimulated mouse peritoneal macrophages causes the synthesis and release of large amounts of ^{3}H-prostaglandins in a time and dose-dependent manner (14). Significant increases in synthesis and release of products are observed as early as thirty minutes after the addition of zymosan and levels continues to increase for at least twenty-four hours (14). The major radioactive oxygenation products were shown to be prostaglandin E$_2$ and 6-keto-prostaglandin F$_{1\alpha}$ (6). Neither prostaglandin F$_{2\alpha}$ or thromboxane B$_2$ were detected in any significant quantities in these experiments. The synthesis of these two major arachidonic acid oxygenation products was found to be inhibited completely by the cyclooxygenase inhibitor indomethacin.

The amounts of prostaglandin E$_2$ synthesized and released was also measured by radioimmunoassay. Cultures containing approximately 5×10^6 resident peritoneal macrophages released more than sixty-fold the baseline level of immunoreactive

TABLE 1

Secretion of Arachidonic Acid Oxygenation Products by Macrophages Elicited by Inflammatory stimuli or exposed to Inflammatory Stimuli in Tissue Culture

Arachidonic acid oxygenation product	Source of mononuclear phagocyte	In vivo Stimulus	In Vitro Stimulus	Reference
PGE	Human peripheral blood monocytes	None	Endotoxin	(20)
	Human intra-uterine contraceptive devices	None	None	(10)
	Guinea pig peritoneum	Mineral oil	None	(11)
		Mineral oil	Lymphokines	(11)
	Rat peritoneum	Casein	Zymosan	(21)
	Mouse peritoneum	None	Zymosan	(6)
		None	Phorbol myristate acetate	(22)
		None	Antibody-coated erythrocytes	(22)
		None	Antigen-antibody complexes	(15)
	Macrophage cell line	None	Endotoxin	(19)
^{3}H- or ^{14}C-PGE$_2$	Mouse peritoneum	None	Zymosan	(6,14)
	Carrageenan granuloma	Carrageenan	None	(23)
PGF$_{2\alpha}$	Human intra-uterine contraceptive devices	None	None	(10)
	Carrageenan granuloma	Carrageenan	None	(25)
^{3}H- or ^{14}C-6-keto PGF$_{1\alpha}$	Mouse peritoneum	None	Antigen-antibody complexes	(15)
	Carrageenan granuloma cell-free homogenates	Carrageenan		(24)
	Carrageenan granuloma slices	Carrageenan	None	(23)
^{14}C-Thromboxane	Cell-free homogenates of macrophages from guinea pig peritoneum	Mineral oil	None	(25)
	Cell-free homogenates of carrageenan granuloma	Carrageenan	None	(24)
Thromboxane B$_2$	Mouse peritoneum	None	Phorbol myristate acetate	(22)

prostaglandin E into their culture medium over a four hour time period when exposed to zymosan (50µg/ml). The amount of immunoreactive prostaglandin E synthesized by such cultures amounted to approximately 400 ng per $5x10^6$ cells in four hours. On the other hand, radioimmunoassay for prostaglandin F in the same experiments showed only baseline levels of this material in both resting cultures and cultures exposed to zymosan (6).

Several other stimuli including antigen-antibody complexes (15), lymphokines (11), endotoxin (16) and phorbol myristate acetate (17) also stimulate prostaglandin synthesis by macrophages.

5. STIMULI LACKING INFLAMMATORY POTENCY DO NOT STIMULATE THE SYNTHESIS OF ARACHIDONIC ACID OXYGENATION PRODUCTS BY MACROPHAGES

In the past we found that stimuli which lack chronic inflammatory potency also failed to cause the selective release of lysosomal acid hydrolases from populations of resident macrophages (12). Such stimuli include latex particles and chrysotile asbestos leached with hydrochloric acid. Populations of resident mouse peritoneal macrophages prelabelled with ^{3}H-arachidonic acid exposed to high concentrations of latex particles also fail to release labeled products (14). The mechanisms underlying this difference in the response of resident mouse peritoneal macrophages to stimuli possessing or lacking chronic inflammatory potency remains unknown. It is pertinent to note that there is no evidence at this time to indicate that the selective release of lysosomal acid hydrolases has any role to play in the initiation of prostaglandin synthesis by resident mouse peritoneal macrophages despite the fact that both classes of products appear to be released from these cells under similar conditions (6).

6. ELICITED MACROPHAGES HAVE A DIMINISHED CAPACITY TO SYNTHESISE ARACHIDONIC OXYGENATION PRODUCTS IN RESPONSE TO INFLAMMATORY STIMULI

Elicited and resident mouse peritoneal macrophages are clearly differentiated by a number of criteria. Elicited cells are generally larger, adhere to and spread on surfaces more rapidly and show greater metabolic activity. In addition they are distinguished from resident macrophages by specific biochemical criteria including their capacity to secrete neutral proteinases, elevated levels of leucine aminopeptidase activity and greatly diminished levels of the plasma membrane ectoenzyme 5'-nucleotidase. Macrophages elicited by thioglycollate broth, *Corynebacterium parvum* or BCG as well as macrophages isolated and cultivated from carrageenan granulomas have a much diminished capacity to synthesise arachidonic acid oxygenation products when compared with resident peritoneal macrophages (18).Resident macrophages give a 42-fold increase in PGE_2 release when exposed for 4 hrs to 50µg/ml zymosan. In contrast, elicited macrophages showed only a 5-fold increase in PGE_2 release when exposed to 300µg/ml of zymosan. A similar loss of reactivity to zymosan in relation to prostaglandin synthesis was found with macrophages from BCG- or *C. parvum*-treated mice. Measurements of the rates of arachidonic acid deacylation from phospholipids of different cell populations show great reductions in arachidonic acid release from elicited cells compared to the release from resident cells. Since arachidonic acid availability is considered rate-limiting for prostaglandin production, this difference could be one factor accounting for diminished prostaglandin production by elicited populations.

7.   CONCLUDING REMARKS

It is now clear that cells of the mononuclear phagocyte system synthesise significant amounts of arachidonic acid oxygenation products. Such production is dependent on both the environment from which the cells are obtained and also on the nature of the stimuli which these cells encounter in their pericellular environment. The physiological and pathological significance of such products is presently the subject of much investigation and speculation (for further discussion see Ref 7 & 8). Progress in this area will depend critically on the further definition of the conditions under which macrophages produce arachidonic acid oxygenation products. That further study is required in this area is attested to by the recent findings that macrophages synthesise hydroxy fatty acid products of the lipoxygenase pathway (9) as well as materials with properties of slow reacting substances of anaphylaxis (19).

ACKNOWLEDGMENT

We wish to thank Mrs. Carolyn Kradjel for her excellent secretarial services.

REFERENCES

1. R. C. Page, P. Davies, A. C. Allison, Int. Rev. Cytol., 52, 119 (1978).

2. P. Davies and R. J. Bonney, J. Reticuloendothel. Soc. 26, 37 (1979).

3. S. Sahn and W. S. Lin, Inflammation 2, 83 (1977).

4. T. P. Stossel, R. J. Mason, and A. L. Smith, J. Clin. Invest. 54, 638 (1974).

5. R. J. Mason, T. P. Stossel, and M. Vaughan, J. Clin. Invest. 51, 2399 (1972).

6. R. J. Bonney, P. D. Wightman, S. Sadowski, F. A. Kuehl Jr. and J. L. Humes, Biochem. J. 176, 433 (1978).

7. P. Davies, R. J. Bonney, J. L. Humes, and F. A. Kuehl Jr., In Proceedings of the Third Leiden Conference on Mononuclear Phagocytes. (R. van Furth, Ed.) Martinus Nijhoff Publishers BV In press.

8. P. Davies, R. J. Bonney, J. L. Humes, F. A. Kuehl Jr., In Regulatory Role of Mononuclear Phagocytes in Immunity. Edited by A. S. Rosenthal and E. R. Unanue, Academic Press, New York In Press.

9. M. Rigaud, J. Durand, J. C. Breton, Biochim. Biophys. Acta 573, 408 (1979).

10. L. Myatt, M. A. Bray, D. A. Gordon and J. Morley, Nature 257, 227 (1975).

11. D. Gordon, M. A. Bray and J. Morley, Nature (London), 262, 401 (1976).

12. H.-U. Schorlemmer, P. Davies, W. Hylton, M. Gugig and A. C. Allison, Brit. J. Exp. Path. 58, 315 (1977).

13. E. C. Keystone, H.-U. Schorlemmer, C. Pope and A. C. Allison, Arth. Rheum. 20, 1396 (1977).

14. J. L. Humes, R. J. Bonney, L. Pelus, M. E. Dahlgren, S. Sadowski, F. A. Kuehl Jr. and P. Davies, Nature (Lond.) 269, 149 (1977).

15. R. J. Bonney, P. Naruns, P. Davies, and J. L. Humes, Prostaglandins. In press.

16. D. L. Rosenstreich, S. N. Vogel, A. R. Jacques, L. M. Wahl and J. J. Oppenheim, J. Immunol. 121, 1664 (1978).

17. J. L. Humes, P. Davies, R. J. Bonney and F. A. Kuehl Jr., Fed. Proc. 37, 1318 (1978).

18. J. L. Humes, S. Burger, M. Galavage, F. A. Kuehl Jr., P. D. Wightman, M. E. Dahlgren, P. Davies, and R. J. Bonney, Submitted for publication, J. Immunol.

19. A. Capron, M. Joseph, J. P. Dessaint, G. Torpier, In Proceedings of the Third Leiden Conference on Mononuclear Phagocytes. (R. van Furth Ed) Martinus Nijhoff Publisher, The Hague. In Press.

20. J. I. Kurland and R. Bockman, J. Exp. Med. 147, 952 (1978).

21. D. Gemsa, M. Seitz, W. Kramer, G. Till and K. Resch, J. Immunol. 120, 1187 (1978).

22. K. Brune, M. Glatt, H. Kalin and H. Peskar, Nature (Lond.) 274, 261 (1978).

23. J. A. Splawinski, B. Wojtaszek, J. Swies and R. J. Gryglewski, Prostaglandins 16, 683 (1978).

24. W.-C. Chang, S.-I. Murota, M. Matsuo and S. Tsurufuji, S., Biochem. Biophys. Res. Commun. 72, 1259 (1976).

25. S.-I. Murota, M. Kawamura and I. Morita, Biochim. Biophys. Acta 528, 507 (1978).

PROSTAGLANDINS AND MACROPHAGES

A.W.Ford-Hutchinson and M.V. Doig, Biochemical Pharmacology
Research Unit, Department of Chemical Pathology, King's College
Hospital Medical School, Denmark Hill, London, SE5 8RX

Introduction

Mononuclear phagocytes are best regarded as multi-function-
al cells playing an important role in the development and maintenance of chronic inflammatory exudates. Thus they eliminate
foreign material such as antigen-antibody complexes; play an
essential role in cell-mediated immunity by functioning as
effector cells and through presentation of antigen to T-lymphocytes; play a cooperative role in antibody production; act as
killer cells producing cytostatic and cytocidal actions upon
tumour and other cells and produce and secrete a large number of
biologically active substances including substantial amounts of
prostaglandins.

The release of prostaglandins by macrophages was first described by Bray, Gordon and Morley (1) who demonstrated, using
bioassay and radioimmunoassay techniques, the release of PGE-
like material from guinea pig exudate cells.   Subsequent studies
have shown that human macrophages release PGE_2 and $PGF_{2\alpha}$, detected by radioimmunoassay, using cells obtained either from implanted intra-uterine contraceptive devices (2) or from human
synovia (3). Murine macrophages have been reported to release
PGE_2, $PGF_{2\alpha}$ and 6-keto-$PGF_{1\alpha}$ identified by thin layer chromatography (4,5), and rat macrophages have been shown to release
PGE_2, $PGF_{2\alpha}$, 6-keto-$PGF_{1\alpha}$ and thromboxane B_2, identified by gas
chromatography-mass spectrometry (6).

It is of considerable importance to quantitate the various
pathways of prostaglandin biosynthesis as individual products
have opposite biological actions. For example PGE_2 and PGI_2 can
inhibit the uptake of thymidine by lymphocytes in response to
mitogen and low doses of cyclo-oxygenase inhibitors, such as indomethacin, can enhance the response (7). On the other hand,
inhibition of thromboxane and lipoxygenase pathways can also inhibit thymidine uptake suggesting that thromboxane A_2 or an uni-
dentified lipoxygenase product can enhance lymphocyte mitogeni-
city (8). The present work describes some quantitative studies
on the release of prostaglandins and thromboxanes by rat macrophages.

Methods

Rat macrophages were obtained from a mixed white cell population by peritoneal lavage. The cells were plated out at a concentration of 2×10^7 cells per $25cm^2$ in Medium 199, pH7.4, containing 5% foetal calf serum, 25 mM N-2 hydroxyethylpiperazine-N'-2-ethane sulphonic acid and antibiotics. The adherent cells were washed at 2h and 24h producing a macrophage population (>95%) as shown by the ability to phagocytose sheep red blood cells, the presence of Fc receptor sites and the presence of granules staining for non-specific esterase. The cells were then cultured for 48h in fresh medium in the presence or absence of rat serum opsonised zymosan ($50\mu g$ ml^{-1}).

At the end of the incubation period, the cells and zymosan were removed by centrifugation, 16, 16-dimethyl PGE_1 and 16, 16-dimethyl $PGF_{2\alpha}$ were added as internal standards and the media was acidified and extracted with diethyl ether. The prostaglandins and thromboxanes in the sample were derivatised to form methyl ester, methoxime, tertiary butyldimethylsilyl ethers. The samples were chromatographed on an OV 101 capillary column interfaced to a VG Micromass 16F mass spectrometer. Quantitative data was obtained by multiple ion detection using the $(M-57)^+$ ions for the prostaglandins and (m/e) 385 for thromboxane B_2.

Results

A quantitative assay system for six products of arachidonic acid metabolism (PGE_1, PGE_2, PGD_2, $PGF_{2\alpha}$, 6-keto-$PGF_{1\alpha}$ and TXB_2) has been developed utilising gas chromatographic separation on a capillary column followed by multiple ion detection using 16, 16-dimethyl analogues of PGE_1 and $PGF_{2\alpha}$ as internal standards. Following extraction from Medium 199, calibration curves were linear (correlation coefficient >0.98) over the range 2 - 300ng for thromboxane B_2, $PGF_{2\alpha}$ and 6-keto-$PGF_{2\alpha}$ and 10-300ng for PGE_1 PGE_2 and PGD_2. The coefficient of variation on repeat extractions was 11%.

Table 1 shows the levels of prostaglandins and thromboxane B_2 detected in media obtained from rat macrophages cultured for 48h in the presence of rat serum-opsonised zymosan. The principal product detected was 6-keto-$PGF_{1\alpha}$, the immediate breakdown product of PGI_2. Lesser amounts of PGE_2, $PGF_{2\alpha}$ and thromboxane B_2 were detected and there was no evidence for the presence of PGE_1 or PGD_2. No significant difference was found in prostaglandin and thromboxane production by the cells in the presence or absence of zymosan which is contrary to previous studies (4). One reason for this may be the length of the culture period (48h). Non-elicited murine macrophages rapidly release lysosomal enzymes such as β-glucuronidase when

TABLE 1

Products of the cyclo-oxygenase pathway from
rat macrophages incubated with zymosan

150-500ng 6-keto-$PGF_{1\alpha}$

Up to 80ng PGE_2

20-80ng TXB_2

Per 2 x 10^7
cells seeded

Up to 40ng $PGF_{2\alpha}$

No evidence for PGE_1 or PGD_2

stimulated by zymosan producing large increases over control
values after 24 hours culture. After three days culture,
however, there is no significant difference between stimulated
and non-stimulated macrophages (9). A similar phenomenon may
be occurring in the case of prostaglandin release by rat macrophages and further studies are being performed to investigate
this point using different time intervals and different stimuli.

These results demonstrate that macrophages produce considerable amounts of 6-keto-$PGF_{1\alpha}$ which implies that these cells
synthesis PGI_2. This is of potential interest in relation
to inflammation as PGI_2 modulates cyclic AMP levels within
macrophages (10) and has also been shown to be a modulator of
vascular permeability responses (11, 12, 13), a potent hyperalgesic agent (14) and a potent inhibitor of lymphocyte transformation (7).

Acknowledgements
     We are grateful to the Science Research Council (M.V.D.) and
Lilly Research, Ltd., for financial support, Dr. Pike of the
Upjohn Co. for prostaglandins and to Dr. W. Dawson and Professor
M.J.H.Smith for help and advice

REFERENCES

(1) M.S.BRAY, D. GORDON and J. MORLEY, Role of prostaglandins
     in reactions in cellular immunity, Brit. J.Pharm., 52,
     453P, (1974).

(2) L.MYATT, M.A. BRAY, D. GORDON and J. MORLEY, Macrophages
     on intra-uterine devices produce prostaglandins, Nature,
     257, 227-228 (1975).

(3) R.A.STURGE, D.B. YATES, D. GORDON, M. FRANCO, W. PAUL,
     M.A. BRAY and J. MORLEY, Prostaglandin production in

arthritis, Ann. Rheum. Dis., $\underline{37}$, 315-320 (1978).

(4) J.L. HUMES, R.J. BONNEY, L. PELUS, M.E. DAHLGREN, S.J.
     SADOWSKI, F.A. KUEHL and P. DAVIES, Macrophages synthesise
     and release prostaglandins in response to inflammatory
     stimuli, Nature, $\underline{269}$, 149-151 (1977).

(5) A. FARZARD, N.S. PENNEYS, A. GHAFFAR, V.A. ZIBOH and J.
     SCHLOSSBERG, PGE_2 and $PGF_2\alpha$ biosynthesis in stimulated
     and non-stimulated peritoneal preparations containing
     macrophages, Prostaglandins, $\underline{14}$, 829-837 (1979).

(6) N.S. CONNOR, E.M. DAVIDSON, M.V. DOIG and A.W. FORD-
     HUTCHINSON, Prostaglandin and thromboxane production by
     rat macrophages, Brit. J. Pharmac., $\underline{66}$ 98P (1979).

(7) D. GORDON, D.C. HENDERSON and J. WESTWICK, The effects of
     prostaglandins E_2 and I_2 on human lymphocyte transformation
     in the presence and absence of inhibitors of prostaglandin
     biosynthesis. Brit. J. Pharmac. In press.

(8) J.P. KELLY, M.C. JOHNSON and C.W. PARKER, Effect of
     inhibitors of arachidonic acid metabolism on mitogenesis
     in human lymphocytes: possible role of thromboxanes and
     products of the lipoxygenase pathway. J. Immunol., $\underline{122}$,
     1563-1571 (1979).

(9) J. SCHNYDER and M. BAGGIOLINI, Role of phagocytosis in the
     activation of macrophages. J.Exp. Med., $\underline{148}$, 1449-1457
     (1978).

(10) R.J. BONNEY, S. BURGER, F.A. KUEHL and J.L. HUMES, Prosta-
     glandin E and prostacyclin elevate cAMP levels in elicited
     but not resident populations of mouse peritoneal macro-
     phages. Advances in Prostaglandin and Thromboxane Research.
     In press.

(11) M.J. PECK and T.J. WILLIAMS, Prostacyclin (PGI_2) potentiates
     bradykinin-induced plasma exudation in the rabbit skin.
     Br. J. Pharmac., $\underline{62}$, 464P (1978).

(12) K. KOMORIYA, H. OHMORI, A. AZUMA, S. KUROZUMI, Y. HASHIMOTO,
     K. NICOLAOU, W. BARNETTE and R. MAGOLDA, Prostaglandin I_2
     as a potentiator of acute inflammation in rats. Prosta-
     glandins, $\underline{15}$, 557-564 (1978).

(13) A.W. FORD-HUTCHINSON, J.R. WALKER, E.M. DAVIDSON and M.J.H.
     SMITH, PGI_2; a potential mediator of inflammation.
     Prostaglandins, $\underline{16}$, 253-258 (1978).

(14) S.H. FERREIRA, M. NAKAMURA, M.S. DE ABROU CASTRO, The
     hyperalgesic effects of prostacyclin and prostaglandin E$_2$
     Prostaglandins. <u>16</u>, 31-37 (1978)

Chapter Four

EFFECTS OF ANTI-INFLAMMATORY DRUGS ON PROSTAGLANDIN
PRODUCTION

PROSTAGLANDIN RELEASE FROM MACROPHAGES: MODULATION BY ANTI-
INFLAMMATORY DRUGS.

K. Brune and K.D. Rainsford
Department of Pharmacology, Biozentrum, University of Basel,
Klingelbergstrasse 70, CH-4056 Basel, Switzerland

B.A. Peskar, Department of Pharmacology, University of
Freiburg, D-78 Freiburg, FRG

I. Why do we measure prostaglandin release from macrophages?
A wealth of information obtained during the last decade indicates that there is no inflammation without prostaglandin (PG) release (1). This indicates that PG's are important mediators of
the inflammatory process or at least obligatory by-products and
consequently useful indicators of this process. On the other
hand, chronic inflammation is always accompanied by infiltrates
of macrophages, and it is widely accepted that these cells are
of major importance for the occurence and propagation of inflammation (2). Since macrophages can be obtained easily, kept
in tissue culture and triggered by inflammatory chemicals to release large quantities of PG's we used these cells to study:
(a) the mechanisms involved in PG-release from macrophages and
(b) the effects of steroidal and non-steroidal anti-inflammatory
drugs on PG-release. The ultimate goal was and still is to establish an in vitro model of inflammation which is more than an
enzyme assay in that it reflects to some extent the important
factor of biodistribution. It is less complex than the in vivo
models which cannot detect drugs which might have anti-inflammatory activity but never reach the target tissue due to poor absorption and pronounced first pass inactivation.

II. Which prostaglandins are released?
Many technical details and results have been published previously (3). In brief, we found that zymosan and antibody-coated erythrocytes are effective triggers of PG-release (10 to 20 times
of controls one hour after their addition). Latex beeds caused
only a delayed and moderate increase of PG-release (2 to 4 times
of controls after 8 hours). This is in agreement with the reported inactivity of these particles in inducing chronic inflammation in vivo (4,5). More effective than these particles
were a variety of well-known and chemically well-defined tumour
promoters which are all highly pro-inflammatory as well (6).
The PG-release induced by these substances correlated with
their pro-inflammatory and tumour-promoting activity in vivo
(6). The amount of PG's released by these compounds reached
a plateau 1 hour after their addition to macrophages and in
our hands, always brought about predominantly the release of
PGE_2, but also substantial amounts of 6-keto $PGF_{1\alpha}$ (the stable
metabolite of PGI_2) and traces of thromboxane TXB_2 and $PGF_{2\alpha}$.
An example of the absolute values is given in the table.

Table: Prostaglandin release from mouse peritoneal macrophages.

Treatment		PG's measured (ng/ml or 10^6 macrophages)		
- 1 hr	0-time	PGE_2	6-keto $F_{1:\alpha}$	TXB_2
Sol_1	Sol_1	3.0±0.3	1.1±0.2	<0.02 -
Sol_1	TPA	16.0±1.1	4.3±0.3	0.58±0.04
Sol_2	TPA	15.4±1.3	3.3±0.2	0.53±0.02
Dexa.	TPA	8.8±1.7**	2.0±0.1**	0.47±0.03**
Indo.	TPA	4.2±0.9**	1.2±0.1**	0.11±0.01**

Mouse peritoneal macrophages obtained and cultivated as described previously (3) were incubated at -1 hr with fresh medium
containing 0.5% solvent (Sol_1 = DMSO; Sol_2 = ethyl alcohol) or
solvent + drug (Sol_2 + dexamethasone final concentration in the
medium 10^{-6}'; Sol_1 + indomethacin, 10^{-7}M). One hour later 12-0-
tetradecanoyl phorbol 13-acetate (TPA) (final concentration
10^{-7}M) in 20 µl DMSO or DMSO alone (control) was added. One
hour after addition of TPA the incubation medium was assayed
for the content of PG's and TXB_2 as described previously (7).
Means and standard deviations of values are given. The values
for TXB_2 were obtained by substracting the concentration of
TXB_2 in the medium before incubation from those obtained thereafter. ** p<0.01 with respect to appropriate controls.

III. How are the prostaglandins released?
An idea about the mechanism(s) involved in PG-release came from
electromicroscopic observations. We found that PG-release induced by antibody-coated erythrocytes coincided with the formation
of a specific type of large vacuoles in macrophages (7). These
vacuoles resemble autophagic vacuoles in that they appear to
contain lysosomal material as well as fragments of the endoplasmic reticulum and occasionally mitochondria. The formation of
these vacuoles and the release of PG's was enhanced by cytocha-
lasin B and inhibited by 2-deoxyglucose although both compounds
reduced phagocytosis (7). Moreover, electron microscopic observations reported by others (8), show that latex beads do not
lead to the formation of similar vacuoles. Finally, tumour promoters induce the rapid formation of a similar type of vacuole
while concanavalin A induces only pinocytotic vacuoles and correspondingly is a very weak stimulator of PG release. These observations were evidence in favour of the suggestion that PG's
were formed in macrophages when lipid membranes containing arachidonic acid, phospholipases from lysosomes and cyclo-oxygenase
from the endoplasmic reticulum are present simultaneously all
in one compartment namely the autophagic vacuole (see fig. 1).

IV. How do anti-inflammatory drugs inhibit prostaglandin release? It is well accepted that the non-steroidal anti-inflammatory (NSAI) drugs block mainly the cyclooxygenase part of the
prostaglandin synthetase enzyme complex. Correspondingly we did
not observe inhibition of vacuole formation in macrophages by
indomethacin during stimulation by tumour promoters or antibody-
coated erythrocytes. On the other hand, it is still a matter
of speculation how glucocorticoids exert their anti-inflammatory
effects. We found, as did others that dexamethasone inhibits
PG-release from macrophages triggered by particles (11) or tumour promoters (13). This effect was apparently independent of
the de novo protein-synthesis (12) and the length of the time
period of pre-incubation of macrophages with dexamethasone (13).
Moreover, it is of relevance that the maximal inhibition of PG-
release possible with dexamethasone was arround 70% (13). These
observations correspond with morphological findings, since we previously found that the reduction of PG release from macrophages
by dexamethasone was paralleled by a reduction of vacuole formation in these cells (13). This observation is further support for
the concept of the mode of action of anti-inflammatory drugs on
PG release from macrophages.

V. What is the relationship between release of PG's and anti-inflammatory activity by NSAI drugs?
It is surprising how well the in vivo anti-inflammatory potency
of a series of non-steroidal drugs correlate with their potency
as inhibitors of prostaglandin release from macrophages in vitro
(fig.2.) The only compound deviating from this correlation is
sulindac which is the pro-drug of sulindac sulfide (10) which itself fits into the correlation.

VI. Conclusions.
In conclusion we like to state that macrophages in culture
appear to be a useful and valid tool to study the molecular and
cellular mechanism(s) being involved in the release of prostaglandins. This system also offers the possibility to study the
modification of pro-inflammatory stimuli in vitro. Finally this
system can be used as a sensitive assay for the detection and
definition of the anti-inflammatory potency of steroid and non-
steroid compounds, with the proviso that drug metabolism/dispo-
sition must be considered.

Acknowledgements
This work was supported by a grant from the Swiss National
Science Foundation (3.588-0.75).

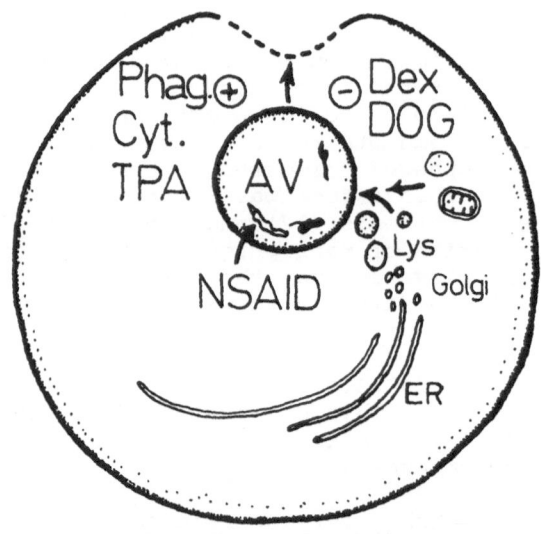

Fig.1 Postulated intracellular mechanisms involved in the for-
       mation of large (autophagic) vacuoles following induction
       by phagocytosis, phagocytosis plus cytochalasin B or che-
       mical irritants (e.g. TPA). Such stimulation denoted by a
       ⊕ effect leads to fusion of lysosomes (LYS) with compo-
       nents of the endoplasmic reticulum (ER)-golgi system (and
       probably other membraneous organelles) so that the resul-
       tant compartment (autophagic vacuole = AV) contains the
       full complement of enzymic machinery for generating large
       quantities of PG's from the abundant membrane-derived phos-
       pholipids, i.e. phospholipases from lysosomes will be pre-
       sent with PG cyclo-oxygenases/isomerases/reductases from
       the ER-golgi-system. Drugs such as dexamethasone which
       block PG production from phospholipid substrates also block
       the formation of autophagic vacuoles (denoted by ϴ effect).
       However, the NSAI drugs such as indomethacin which only
       block the cyclo-oxygenase pathway do not block the for-
       mation of AV's.

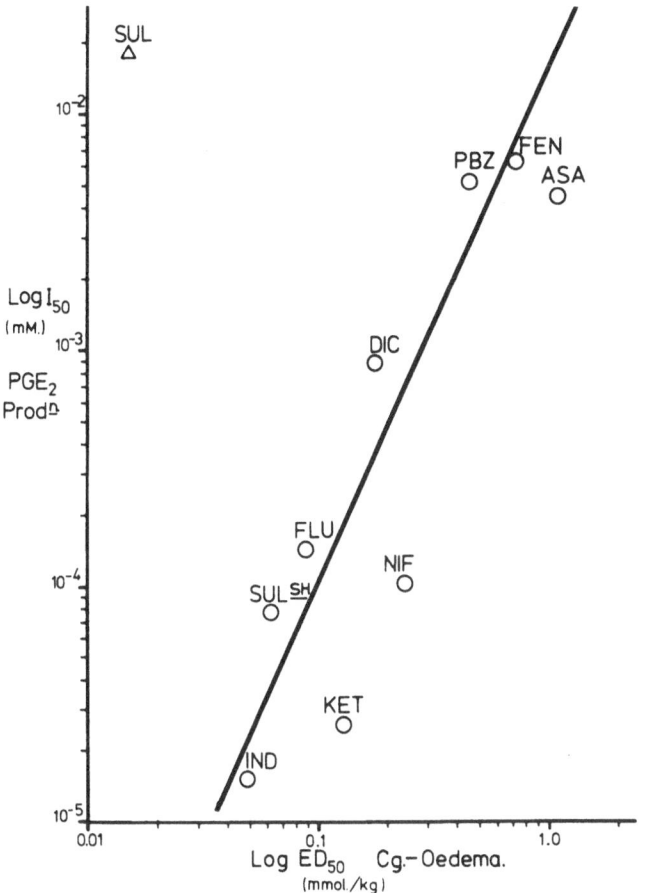

Fig.2 Correlation between inhibition of macrophage prostaglan-
        din E_2 production and anti-inflammatory activity for a
        series of acidic NSAI drugs. A significant correlation
        ($r = 0.86$) was obtained when the pro-drug sulindac was
        excluded from the statistical analysis. This correlation
        is, however, maintained if sulindas sulphide (the pharma-
        cologically active metabolite) is included in the ana-
        lysis, thus illustrating the importance of drug metabo-
        lism in relation to effects on PG-production. Data on
        anti-inflammatory activity (carrageenin-induced oedema
        in rats) was derived from refs. 10, 14, 15 and was self-
        consistent in that data of standard drugs (e.g. aspirin,
        indomethacin) agreed well. Drug abbreviations:
        ASA = aspirin, DIC = diclofenac, FEN = fenclofenac,
        FLU = flufenamic acid, IND = indomethacin, KET = keto-
        profen, NIF = niflumic acid, PBZ = phenylbutazone,
        SUL = sulindac, SUL-SH = sulindac sulfide.

REFERENCES

(1)   S.H. FERREIRA and J.R. VANE, Mode of action of anti-in-
      flammatory agents which are prostaglandin synthetase inhi-
      bitors. In Anti-inflammatory Drugs (Eds. J.R. Vane and
      S.H. Ferreira). Handbook of Experimental Pharmacology,
      Vol. 50/II. pp. 348-398. Springer-Verlag, Heidelberg (1979).

(2)   P. DAVIES and A.C. ALLISON. The release of hydrolytic en-
      zymes from phagocytic and other cells participating in
      acute and chronic inflammation. In Inflammation (Eds. J.R.
      Vane and S.H. Ferreira). Handbook of Experimental Pharmaco-
      logy, Vol. 50/I. pp. 267-294. Springer-Verlag, Heidelberg
      (1979).

(3)   M. GLATT, H. KÄLIN, K. WAGNER and K. BRUNE. Prostaglandin
      release from macrophages: An assay system for anti-inflamma-
      tory drugs in vitro. Agents and Actions 7, 321-326 (1977).

(4)   J.L. HUMES, R.J. BONNEY, L. PELUS, M.E. DAHLGREN,
      S.J. Sadowski, F.A. KUEHL, jr. and P. DAVIES. Macrophages
      synthesize and release prostaglandins in response to in-
      flammatory stimuli. Nature 269, 149-151 (1977).

(5)   H.-U. SCHORLEMMER, P. DAVIES, W. HYLTON, M. GUGIG and
      A.C. ALLISON. The selective release of lysosomal hydrolases
      from mouse peritoneal macrophages by stimuli of chronic
      inflammation. Br. J. Exp. Path. 58, 315-320 (1977).

(6)   K. BRUNE, H. KÄLIN, R. SCHMIDT and E. HECKER. Inflammatory,
      tumour initiating and promoting activities of polycyclic
      aromatic hydrocarbons and diterpene esters in mouse skin
      as compared with their prostaglandin releasing potency in
      vitro. Cancer Lett. 4, 333-342 (1978).

(7)   K. BRUNE, M. GLATT, H. KÄLIN and B.A. PESKAR. Pharmacolo-
      gical control of prostaglandin and thromboxane release from
      macrophages. Nature 274, 261-263 (1978).

(8)   R.M. STEINMAN and Z.A. COHN. Mononuclear phygocytes. In:
      The Inflammatory Process (Eds. B.W. Zweifach, L. Grand
      and R.T. McCluskey) pp.449-510 (Academic Press, New York
      (1979).

(9)   K.A. CHANDRABOSE, E.G. LAPETINA, C.J. SCHMITGES,
      M.J. SIEGEL and P. CUATRECASAS. Action of corticosteroids
      in regulation of prostaglandin biosynthesis in cultured
      fibroblasts. Proc. Nat. Acad. Sci. 75, 214-217 (1978).

(10) T.Y. SHEN and C.A. WINTER. Chemical and biological studies
      on indomethacin, sulindac and their analogs. Adv. in Drug
      Res. 12, 89-245 (1977).

(11) M.A. BRAY and D. GORDON. Prostaglandin production by macro-
     phages and the effect of anti-inflammatory drugs. Br. J.
     Pharmac. 63, 635-642 (1978).

(12) K. BRUNE and K. WAGNER. The effects of protein/nucleic
     acid synthesis inhibitors on the inhibition of prostaglan-
     din release from macrophages by dexamethasone. In:
     Arachidonic acid metabolism in inflammation and thrombosis
     (Eds. K. Brune and M. Baggiolini) Agents and Actions
     Suppl. AAS4. pp 73-77, Birkhauser-Verlag, Stuttgart (1979).

(13) K. BRUNE, H. KÄLIN, K.D. RAINSFORD and K. WAGNER. Dexa-
     methasone inhibits the release of prostaglandins and the
     formation of autophagic vacuoles from stimulated macropha-
     ges. Advances in Prostaglandin and Thromboxane Research 5,
     in press.

(14) D.C. ATKINSON and E.C. LEACH. Anti-inflammatory and related
     properties of 2-(2,4-dichlorophenoxy)phenyl acetic acid
     (Fenclofenac). Agents and Actions 6, 657-666 (1976).

(15) J.G. LOMBARDINO, I.G. OTTERNESS and E.H. WISEMAN. Acidic
     anti-inflammatory agents - correlations of some physical,
     pharmacological and clinical data. Arzneim.-Forsch. 25,
     1629-1635 (1975).

ARACHIDONIC ACID METABOLISM IN INFLAMMATION AND THE MODE OF ACTION OF ANTI-INFLAMMATORY DRUGS

G.A. Higgs, K.E. Eakins, S. Moncada and J.R. Vane
Dept. of Prostaglandin Research, Wellcome Research Laboratories, Langley Court, Beckenham, Kent BR3 3BS, U.K.

The products of arachidonic acid metabolism were first implicated in the inflammatory response in 1969, when Piper and Vane (1) demonstrated the release of "rabbit aorta contracting substance" (RCS) and of prostaglandins during anaphylaxis and Willis (2) showed the release of prostaglandins in carrageenin-induced inflammatory exudates in the rat. In the following years, prostaglandins were detected in numerous inflammatory conditions in animals and man and they were found to have potent vasodilator, hyperalgesic and pyretic properties. By 1977, the evidence to support the theory that prostaglandins are involved in inflammation was so extensive that Ryan and Majno (3), in their review of acute inflammation, grouped prostaglandins with vasoactive amines and kinins as the most likely chemical mediators of the vascular resonses in inflammation. A key step in the development of the idea that prostaglandins are inflammatory mediators was the discovery in 1971 that aspirin and other non-steroid anti-inflammatory drugs selectively inhibited prostaglandin biosynthesis (4-6). This led Vane (4) to propose that inhibition of prostaglandin synthesis explains the therapeutic and toxic effects of aspirin-like drugs. The contribution of prostaglandins to the inflammatory process and the mode of action of anti-inflammatory drugs which are prostaglandin synthetase inhibitors has been comprehensively discussed by Ferreira and Vane (7).

In recent years the metabolic transformations of arachidonic acid have come under close biochemical scrutiny. Cyclic endoperoxides have been identified as unstable intermediates in the synthesis of prostaglandins (8). As precursors of the stable prostaglandins, thromboxanes (9) and prostacyclin (10), they occupy a pivotal position in the cyclo-oxygenase pathway of arachidonic acid oxygenation. In 1974, the observation that platelets contain a lipoxygenase (11,12) demonstrated that there is an alternative route of fatty acid oxygenation giving rise to a series of hydroperoxy and hydroxy acids. In this paper, we consider the possible significance of these newly discovered metabolites and the effects that anti-inflammatory drugs might have upon their production.

CYCLO-OXYGENASE PRODUCTS

1. Cyclic Endoperoxides

The cyclic endoperoxides (PGG_2 and PGH_2) are generated from arachidonic acid by a dioxygenase reaction with the incorporation of molecular oxygen (8). PGG_2 and PGH_2 potentiate carrageenin-induced oedema (13) and PGH_2 enhances the effects of other mediators in cutaneous inflammation (14). The activity of the endoperoxides in vivo may be due to conversion to other substances such as PGE_2 which has a similar action.

It has been suggested that some inflammatory effects are due to the generation of a free oxygen radical during the conversion of PGG_2 to PGH_2 (15). The radical scavenger MK447, which inhibits carrageenin-induced oedema, facilitates the conversion of PGG_2 to PGH_2 in vitro, without preventing the synthesis of stable prostaglandins. Also PGH_2 is less active in producing pain and oedema than PGG_2 (13,16). However, PGG_2 is not as potent as PGE_2 in inducing exudation in rabbit skin (17) or causing oedema in the rat paw (18).

2.   Thromboxanes

In 1969, Piper and Vane (1) detected a labile substance in the effluent of isolated perfused lungs during anaphylaxis which could not be matched by a known prostaglandin. This activity is now known to be due to a mixture of endoperoxides and thromboxanes (9,19). The thromboxanes are non-prostanoate structures which are derived from PGG_2 and PGH_2 (9). There are no reports on the effects of thromboxane A_2 (TXA_2) in inflammation but it is a potent aggregator of platelets and a vasoconstrictor (20). Thromboxane generating enzymes have been detected in platelets (21) polymorphonuclear leukocytes (PMNs; 22), macrophages (23,24) and granuloma tissues (25) and these cells may contribute to the thromboxane activity found in inflammatory exudates (26,27). TXB_2, the stable breakdown product of TXA_2 is chemotactic for mouse PMNs (28) and may, therefore, be involved in the characteristic accumulation of cells at an inflammatory site. TXB_2 is not, however, chemotactic for human leukocytes (29).

3.   Prostacyclin

In blood vessel walls, cyclic endoperoxides are converted to another unstable substance, prostacyclin (PGI_2; 10), which has opposing biological activities to TXA_2; it inhibits platelet aggregation and is vasodilator (30). The stable break-down product of prostacyclin, 6-oxo-$PGF_{1\alpha}$ (31), has been detected in inflammatory exudates (27,32). The source of prostacyclin production in inflammation may be blood vessels, macrophages (33) or granuloma tissue (32). Prostacyclin induces rat-paw oedema, enhances carrageenin-induced oedema (34,35) and potentiates bradykinin-induced plasma exudation in rabbit skin (36). Prostacyclin is 3-5 times less potent than PGE_2 in inducing oedema in the rat paw or rabbit skin, but is approximately 80 times more active than PGE_2 as a vasodilator in the hamster cheek pouch microcirculation (37). Prostacyclin also causes hyperalgesia (34,38) and there is evidence that PGI_2 rather than PGE_2 is the endogenous mediator of carrageenin-induced hyperalgesia in the rat foot (38). The presence of comparable concentrations of PGE_2 and 6-oxo-$PGF_{1\alpha}$ in inflammatory exudates (27) indicates that both PGE_2 and prostacyclin contribute to the vasodilatation and hyperalgesia seen in acute inflammation.

Prostacyclin elevates cyclic AMP (39) and adenyl cyclase stimulation is associated with anti-inflammatory effects. PGE_1-stimulated increases in PMN cyclic AMP are related to inhibition of the motility of these cells (40). Prostacyclin inhibits chemotaxis in vitro (41) and prevents the characteristic margination and adherence of leukocytes to inflamed blood vessel walls (42). Thus, prostacyclin, while mediating the vascular and hyperalgesic responses in acute inflammation, could reduce the migration of leukocytes in the chronic phase. In this respect it is interesting that total leukocyte numbers in 8-day inflammatory exudates are at their highest when 6-oxo-$PGF_{1\alpha}$ concentrations are at their lowest (27).

LIPOXYGENASE PRODUCTS

1. Hydroxy acids

An alternative pathway of arachidonic acid oxygenation is the platelet lipoxygenase which generates 12-L-hydroxy-eicosatetraenoic acid (12-HETE) during aggregation (11,12). 12-HETE is a potent chemotactic agent for human PMNs (43,44) and a lipid function derived from E. Coli has the same chemotactic properties and chromatographic mobility as 12-HETE (45). Platelet lipoxygenases also produce tri-hydroxy acids (THETAs) from arachidonic acid (46) and these too have chemotactic properties (47).

It is unlikely, however, that platelets play an important role in leukocyte migration in vivo as cell numbers are not significantly reduced in inflammatory exudates from thrombocytopenic rats (48). Furthermore, the inflammatory response proceeds virtually unimpaired in the absence of circulating platelets (49). 12-HETE has been detected in inflamed skin (50) and leucocytes are a possible source of chemotatic lipoxygenase products in inflammation. Rabbit PMNs generate 5-HETE from arachidonic acid (51) and rat peritoneal leukocytes produce a mixture of 11-HETE and 12-HETE (52,53). 5-HETE is more potent than 12-HETE in attracting human leukocytes (54) and the chemotactic properties of these hydroxy acids are comparable with those of the complement fraction C5a (44). Production of HETEs by leukocytes could, therefore, represent a local control mechanism for the accumulation of inflammatory cells.

The cyclo-oxygenase product 12-L-hydroxyheptadecatrienoic acid (HHT; 11) has less chemotactic activity for PMNs than 12-HETE (29) but it stimulates chemokinesis in T-lymphocytes whereas 12-HETE, PGE_2, $PGF_{2\alpha}$ and TXB_2 do not have this activity (55).

2. Leukotrienes

In their investigation of leukocyte lipoxygenases, Borgeat and Samuelsson have detected the generation of a di-hydroxy acid, 5,12-HETE, from arachidonic acid (56). They have now shown that 5,12-HETE is one of a family of related compounds which they have named leukotrienes (57). Leukotriene C is similar in biological properties to slow reacting substance of anaphylaxis (SRS-A). The importance of the leukotrienes in inflammation is not yet known but it is possible that they are involved in the vascular or cellular components of some types of inflammatory response.

ANTI-INFLAMMATORY DRUGS

1. Cyclo-oxygenase inhibitors

Stable prostaglandins are present in sufficient concentrations in most inflammatory conditions to cause and enhance the cardinal signs of inflammation and the selective inhibition of prostaglandin biosynthesis accounts for the anti-inflammatory properties of drugs such as indomethacin and the salicylates (7). In addition, cyclo-oxygenase inhibition prevents the vasodilatation and hyperalgesia mediated by prostacyclin (34,38).

Inhibition of prostaglandin, TXB_2 and HHT production may impair leukocyte function in inflammation but leukocyte migration is not reduced by doses of indomethacin which just abolish prostaglandin synthesis (58). Non-steroid cyclo-oxygenase inhibitors give good symptomatic relief of pain and swelling in acute and chronic inflammation but it is generally stated that in chronic inflammation the underlying cause of the disease proceeds unchecked during prolonged administration of these drugs. Lipoxygenase products are more potent chemotactic agents than cyclo-oxygenase products (29) and failure to inhibit lipoxygenase may explain why drugs like indomethacin and aspirin have relatively weak effects on leukocyte migration. In fact, indomethacin and aspirin potentiate lipoxygenase activity in vitro (11) possibly through a diversion of substrate. This may explain why cyclo-oxygenase inhibitors enhance leukocyte migration in vivo (59-61). Higher doses cause a reduction in migrating cells (58,59,61) and it is possible, therefore, that low doses selectively inhibit cyclo-oxygenase, while higher doses prevent both pathways of arachidonic acid oxygenation. In the clinic, low doses of cyclo-oxygenase inhibitors are chosen in an attempt to minimise toxic effects. These doses would be expected to give symptomatic relief through inhibition of prostaglandin synthesis but the more chronic, leukocyte-mediated inflammatory effects may be enhanced.

2.   Steroids

The anti-inflammatory steroid, dexamethasone, does not inhibit cyclo-oxygenase or lipoxygenase in vitro (62) but prevents prostaglandin production in the rabbit mesenteric bed (63) and in isolated synovial cells in culture (64). The relative potency of the corticosteroids in blocking the release of arachidonic acid from perfused guinea-pig lungs is very similar to their relative anti-inflammatory potency (65) and it now appears that steroids induce the release of a substance which inhibits phospholipase A_2 (66). Such an activity would prevent the release of arachidonic acid from phospholipids and may account for the "membrane stabilization" effects associated with steroids. Reduced availability of arachidonic acid would lead to a decrease in both cyclo-oxygenase and lipoxygenase products. The indirect inhibition of lipoxygenase may contribute to the effects of steroids on leukocyte migration. This would explain why dexamethasone is equi-active in reducing prostaglandin concentrations and leukocyte numbers in inflammatory exudates (62).

3.   Dual cyclo-oxygenase and lipoxygenase inhibitors

Two types of compound inhibit both pathways of arachidonic acid oxygenation; these are substrate analogues such as 5,8,11,14 eicosatetraynoic acid (TYA; 11) and a series of phenyl-pyrazolines (62,67,68). TYA prevents prostaglandin production in vivo but does not affect leukocyte migration (58). This may be because TYA inhibits platelet lipoxygenase but does not inhibit leukocyte lipoxygenase (51). BW755C (3-amino-1-[m-(trifluoromethyl)-phenyl]-2-pyrazoline) inhibits lung (69), platelet (62) and leukocyte (52) lipoxygenases in vitro and, like dexamethasone, causes a reduction in prostaglandin concentrations and leukocyte numbers in vivo (62). BW755C does not enhance leukocyte numbers at any dose and reverses the indomethacin-induced increase in leukocyte numbers in inflammatory exudates (61).

A compound which prevents both pathways of arachidonic acid metabolism has the advantage over selective cyclo-oxygenase inhibitors of avoiding potentiation of lipoxygenase and of having a greater effect in reducing leukocyte migration at doses which inhibit prostaglandin synthesis. A dual inhibitor could also have advantages by being free of the complicating systemic side effects associated with anti-inflammatory steroids.

The potential therapeutic importance of dual inhibitors is also indicated in the treatment of other diseases. Indomethacin potentiates the release of SRS-A and histamine from perfused lungs during anaphylactic challenge, while an analogue of

BW755C does not have this effect (67). It is possible that the development of a drug which is equi-active in inhibiting both enzymes may be the next step in the evolution of non-steroid drugs for the treatment of chronic inflammation and bronchoconstriction.

REFERENCES

1. Piper, P.J. and Vane, J.R. Release of additional factors in anaphylaxis and its antagonism by anti-inflammatory drugs. Nature, 223:29 (1969).

2. Willis, A.L. Release of histamine, kinin and prostaglandins during carrageenin-induced inflammation of the rat. In: Prostaglandins, peptides and amines. (P. Mantegazza and E.W. Horton, eds.) Academic Press, London, 1969, p.65.

3. Ryan, G.B. and Majno, G. Acute inflammation. Am. J. Path., 86:184 (1977).

4. Vane, J.R. Inhibition of prostaglandin synthesis as a mechanism of action for the aspirin-like drugs. Nature, 231:232 (1971).

5. Smith, J.B. and Willis, A.L. Aspirin selectively inhibits prostaglandin production in human platelets. Nature, 231:235 (1971).

6. Ferreira, S.H., Moncada, S. and Vane, J.R. Indomethacin and aspirin abolish prostaglandin release from the spleen. Nature, 231:237 (1971).

7. Ferreira, S.H. and Vane, J.R. Mode of action of anti-inflammatory agents which are prostaglandin synthetase inhibitors. In: Anti-inflammatory drugs, eds. J.R. Vane and S.H Ferreira, Springer-Verlag (1979).

8. Hamberg, M., Svensson, J., Wakabayashi, T. and Samuelsson, B. Isolation and structure of two prostaglandin endoperoxides that cause platelet aggregation. Proc. Nat. Acad. Sci., 71:345 (1974).

9. Hamberg, M., Svensson, J. and Samuelsson, B. Thromboxanes: A new group of biologically active compounds derived from prostaglandin endoperoxides. Proc. Nat. Acad. Sci., 72:2994 (1975).

10. Moncada, S., Gryglewski, R.J., Bunting, S. and Vane, J.R. An enzyme isolated from arteries transforms prostaglandin endoperoxides to an unstable substance that inhibits platelet aggregation. Nature, 263:663 (1976).

11. Hamberg, M. and Samuelsson, B. Prostaglandin endoperoxides. Novel transformations of arachidonic acid in human platelets. Proc. Nat. Acad. Sci., 71:3400 (1974).

12. Nugteren, D.A. Arachidonate lipoxygenase in blood platelets. Biochim. Biophys. Acta., 380:299 (1975).

13. Vane, J.R. Prostaglandins as mediators of inflammation. In: Advances in prostaglandin and thromboxane research, edited by B. Samuelsson and R. Paoletti, Vol 2: p. 791, Raven Press, New York (1976).

14. Hagermark, O., Strandberg, K. and Hamberg, M. Potentiating effects of prostaglandin E_2 and the prostaglandin endoperoxide PGH_2 on cutaneous responses in man. J. Invest. Derm., 66:266P (1976).

15. Kuehl, F.A., Humes, J.L., Egan, R.W., Ham, E.A., Beveridge, G.C. and Van Arman, C.G. Role of prostaglandin endoperoxide PGG_2 in inflammatory processes. Nature, 265:170 (1977).

16. Willis, A.L., Vane, F.M., Kuhn, D.C., Scott, C.G. and Petrin, M. An endoperoxide aggregator (LASS) formed in platelets in response to thrombotic stimuli. Prostaglandins, 8:453 (1974).

17. Williams T.J. and Peck, M.J. Role of prostaglandin-mediated vasodilatation in inflammation. Nature, 270:530 (1977).

18. Moncada, S. New developments in the knowledge of arachidonic acid metabolic products in inflammation. Eur. J. Rheum. Inflam., 2:90 (1979).

19. Moncada, S. and Vane, J.R. The discovery of prostacyclin: A fresh insight into arachidonic acid metabolism. In: Biochemical aspects of prostaglandins and thromboxanes, ed. N. Kharasch and J. Fried, Academic Press, p. 155 (1977).

20. Dusting, G.J., Moncada, S. and Vane, J.R. Vascular actions of arachidonic acid and its metabolites in perfused mesenteric and femoral beds of the dog. Eur. J. Pharmac., 49:65 (1978).

21. Needleman, P., Moncada, S., Bunting, S., Vane, J.R., Hamberg, M. and Samuelsson, B. Identification of an enzyme in platelet microsomes which generates thromboxane A_2 from prostaglandin endoperoxides. Nature, 261:558 (1976).

22. Higgs, G.A., Bunting, S., Moncada, S. and Vane, J.R. Polymorphonuclear leukocytes produce thromboxane A_2-like activity during phagocytosis. Prostaglandins, 12:749 (1976).

23. Brune, K., Glatt, M. and Kalin, H. Pharmacological control of prostaglandin and thromboxane release from macrophages. Nature, 274:261 (1978).

24. Murota, S-I., Kawamura, M. and Morita, I. Transformation of arachidonic acid into thromboxane B_2 by the homogenates of activated macrophages. Biochim. Biophys. Acta. 528:507 (1978).

25. Chang, W.C., Murota, S-I. and Tsurufuji, S. Thromboxane B_2 transformed from arachidonic acid in carrageenin-induced granuloma. Prostaglandins, 13:17 (1977).

26. Trang, L.E., Granstrom, E. and Lovgren, O. Levels of prostaglandin $F_{2\alpha}$ and E_2 and thromboxane B_2 in joint fluid in rheumatoid arthritis. Scand. J. Rheum. 6:151 (1977).

27. Higgs, G.A. and Salmon, J.A. Cyclo-oxygenase products in carrageenin-induced inflammation. Prostaglandins, 17:737 (1979).

28. Boot, J.R., Dawson, W. and Kitchen, E.A. The chemotactic activity of thromboxane B_2: A possible role in inflammation. J. Physiol., 257:47P (1976).

29. Goetzl, E.J. and Gorman, R.R. Chemotactic and chemokinetic stimulation of human eosinophil and neutrophil polymorphonuclear leukocytes by 12-L-hydroxy-5,8,10-heptadecatrienoic acid (HHT). J. Immunol., 120:526 (1978).

30. Armstrong, J.M., Chapple, D., Dusting, G.J., Hughes, R., Moncada, S. and Vane, J.R. Cardiovascular actions of prostacyclin (PGI_2) in chloralose anaesthetized dogs. Br. J. Pharmac., 61:136P (1977).

31. Johnson, R.A., Morton, D.R., Kinner, J.H., Gorman, R.R., McGuire, J.C., Sun, F.F., Whittaker, N., Bunting, S., Salmon, J.A., Moncada, S. and Vane, J.R. The chemical structure of prostaglandin X (prostacyclin). Prostaglandins, 12:915 (1976).

32. Chang, W.C., Murota, S-I., Matsuo, M. and Tsurufuji, S. A new prostaglandin transformed from arachidonic acid in carrageenin-induced granuloma. Biochem. Biophys. Res. Commun., 72:1259 (1976).

33. Humes, J.L., Bonney, R.J., Pelus, L., Dahlgren, M.E., Sadowski, S.J., Kuehl, F.A. and Davies, P. Macrophages synthesise and release prostaglandin in response to inflammatory stimuli. Nature, 269:149 (1977).

34. Higgs, E.A., Moncada, S. and Vane, J.R. Inflammatory effects of prostacyclin (PGI_2) and 6-oxo-$PGF_{1\alpha}$ in the rat paw. Prostaglandins, 16:153 (1978).

35. Komoriya, K., Ohmori, H., Azuma, A., Kurozumi, S., Hashimoto, Y., Nicolaou, K.C., Barnette, W.E. and Magolda, R.L. Prostaglandin I_2 as a potentiator of acute inflammation in rats. Prostaglandins, 15:557 (1978).

36. Peck, M.J. and Williams, T.J. Prostacyclin (PGI_2) potentiates bradykinin-induced plasma exudation in rabbit skin. Br. J. Pharmac., 62:464P (1978).

37. Higgs, G.A., Cardinal, D.C., Moncada, S. and Vane, J.R. Microcirculatory effects of prostacyclin (PGI_2) in the hamster cheek pouch. Microvascular Res., In press (1979).

38. Ferreira, S.H., Nakamura, M. and Abreu Castro, M.S. The hyperalgesic effects of prostacyclin and PGE_2. Prostaglandins, 16:31 (1978).

39. Tateson, J.E., Moncada, S. and Vane, J.R. Effects of prostacyclin (PGX) on cyclic AMP concentrations in human platelets. Prostaglandins, 13:389 (1977).

40. Rivkin, I., Rosenblatt, J. and Becker, E.L. The role of cyclic AMP in the chemotactic responsiveness and spontaneous motility of rabbit peritoneal neutrophils. J. Immunol., 115:1126 (1974).

41. Weksler, B.B., Knapp, J.M. and Jaffe, E.A. Prostacyclin (PGI_2) synthesised by cultured endothelial cells modulates polymorphonuclear leukocyte function. Blood, 50(5)Suppl. 1, p.287 (1977).

42. Higgs, G.A., Moncada, S. and Vane, J.R. Prostacyclin reduces the number of 'slow moving' leukocytes in hamster cheek pouch venules. J. Physiol., 280:55P (1978).

43. Turner, S.R., Tainer, J.A. and Lynn, W.S. Biogenesis of chemotactic molecules by the arachidonate lipoxygenase system of platelets. Nature, 257:680 (1975).

44. Goetzl, E.J., Woods, J.M. and Gorman, R.R. Stimulation of human eosinophil and neutrophil polymorphonuclear leukocyte chemotaxis and random migration by 12-L-Hydroxy-5,8,10,14-eicosatetraenoic acid. J. Clin. Invest. 59:179 (1977).

45. Tainer, J.A., Turner, S.R. and Lynn, W.S. New aspects of chemotaxis: specific target cell attraction by lipid and lipoprotein fractions of Escherichia Coli chemotactic factor. Am. J. Path., 81:401 (1975).

46. Jones, R.L., Kerry, P.J., Poyser, N.L., Walker, I.C. and Wilson, N.H. The identification of trihydroxyeicosatrienoic acids as products from the incubation of arachidonic acid with washed blood platelets. Prostaglandins, 16:583 (1978).

47. Jones, R.L., Walker, I.C. and Wilson, N.H. Epoxy-hydroxy and trihydroxy compounds identified as incubation products of arachidonic acid with washed blood platelets. Proceedings of the Fourth International Prostaglandin Conference Washington, (1979).

48. Higgs, G.A. Prostaglandins, polymorphonuclear leukocytes and their contribution to the inflammatory process. Ph.D. Thesis (1976).

49. Ubatuba, F.B., Harvey, E.A. and Ferreira, S.H. Are platelets important in inflammation? Agents and Actions, 5:31 (1975).

50. Hammerstrom, S., Hamberg, M., Samuelsson, B., Duells, E.A., Stawski, M. and Voorhees, J.J. Increased concentrations of non-esterified arachidonic acid, 12L-hydroxy 5,8,10,14-eicosatetraenoic acid, prostaglandin E_2 and prostaglandin $F_{2\alpha}$ in epidermis of psoriasis. Proc. Nat. Acad. Sci., USA, 72:5130 (1975).

51. Borgeat, P., Hamberg, M. and Samuelsson, B. Transformation of arachidonic acid and homo-γ-linolenic acid by polymorphonuclear leukocytes. J. Biol. Chem., 251:7816 (1976).

52. Higgs, G.A., Eakins, K.E., Russell-Smith, N., Mugridge, K.G. and Moncada, S. Inhibition of rat-leukocyte lipoxygenase by BW755C. Proceedings of the Fourth International Prostaglandin Conference, Washington, (1979).

53. McGuire, J.C. and Sun, F.F. Metabolism of arachidonic acid and prostaglandin endoperoxide by assorted leukocytes. Proceedings of the Fourth International Prostaglandin Conference, Washington, (1979).

54. Goetzl, E.J., Brash, A.R., Oates, J.A. and Hubbard, W.C. Functional determinants of the monohydroxy eicosatetraenoic acids (HETEs) which stimulate human neutrophil and eosinophil chemotaxis. Fed. Proc., 38:1085 (1979).

55. McCarty, J. and Goetzl, E.J. Stimultion of human T-lymphocyte chemokinesis by arachidonic acid. Cell Immunol. 43:103 (1979).

56.   Borgeat, P. and Samuelsson, B. Transformations of arachidonic acid by rabbit polymorphonuclear leukocytes. J. Biol. Chem., 254:2643 (1979).

57.   Borgeat, P. and Samuelsson, B. Metabolism of arachidonic acid in human polymorphonuclear leukocytes: Effects of the Ionophore A23187. Proceedings of the Fourth International Prostaglandin Conference, Washington, (1979).

58.   Walker, J.R., Smith, M.J.H. and Ford-Hutchinson, A.W. Anti-inflammatory drugs, Prostaglandins and leukocyte migration.   Agents & Actions, 6:602 (1976).

59.   Adams, S.S., Burrows, C.A., Skeldon, N. and Yates, D.B.   Inhibition of prostaglandin synthesis and leukocyte migration by flurbiprofen. Current Med. Res., 5:11 (1977).

60.   Srinivasan, B.D., Kulkarni, P.S. and Eakins, K.E.   Characterization of chemotactic factors in corneal wound healing. Proceedings of the Fourth International Prostaglandin Conference, Washington, (1979).

61.   Eakins, K.E., Higgs, G.A., Mugridge, K.G., Moncada, S. and Vane, J.R. Low doses of indomethacin or the salicylates enhance leukocyte migration in vivo. In press (1979).

62.   Higgs, G.A., Flower, R.J. and Vane, J.R.   A new approach to anti-inflammatory drugs. Biochem. Pharm., 28:1959 (1979).

63.   Gryglewski, R.J., Panczenko, B., Korbut, R., Grodzinska, L. and Ocetkiewicz, A.   Corticosteroids inhibit prostaglandin release from perfused lungs of sensitized guinea-pigs. Prostaglandins, 10:343 (1975).

64.   Hong, S.L. and Levine, L. Inhibition of arachidonic acid release from cells as the biochemical action of anti-inflammatory corticosteroids.   Proc. Nat. Acad. Sci., USA, 73:1730 (1976).

65.   Nijkamp, F.P., Flower, R.J., Moncada, S. and Vane, J.R. Partial purification of RCS-RF (rabbit aorta contracting substance releasing factor) and inhibition of its activity by anti-inflammatory steroids. Nature, 263:479 (1976).

66.   Flower, R.J. and Blackwell, G.J.   Anti-inflammatory steroids induce biosynthesis of a phospholipase A_2 inhibitor which prevents prostaglandin generation. Nature, 278:456 (1979).

67.   Adcock, J.J., Garland, L.G., Moncada, S. and Salmon, J.A. The mechanism of enhancement by fatty acid hydroperoxides of anaphylactic mediator release. Prostaglandins, 16:179 (1978).

68.   Blackwell, G.J. and Flower, R.J. 1-Phenyl-3-pyrazolidone: an inhibitor of cyclo-oxygenase and lipoxygenase pathways in lung and platelets. Prostaglandins, 16:417 (1978).

69.   Higgs, G.A., Copp, F.C., Denyer, C.V., Flower, R.J., Tateson, J.E., Vane, J.R. and Walker, J.M.G. Reduction of leukocyte migration by a cyclo-oxygenase and lipoxygenase inhibitor. Proceedings of the 7th International Congress of Pharmacology, Abstract 843, Paris, (1978).

SOME MEDICINAL CHEMICAL ASPECTS OF
PROSTAGLANDIN SYNTHESIS INHIBITORS

T. Y. Shen

Membrane and Arthritis Research
Merck Sharp and Dohme Research Laboratories
Rahway, New Jersey 07065 U.S.A.

1. INTRODUCTION

Since the original observation by Vane and his associates (1) that aspirin and indomethacin are inhibitors of prostaglandin biosynthesis in 1971, numerous compounds have been reported to possess similar properties. Several comprehensive reviews (2,3) of their structure-activity relationships, mainly in terms of cyclooxygenase inhibition and antiinflammatory potency in animal models have been published. In recent years, the possible contribution of various biochemical and pharmacodynamic aspects to the overall efficacy and tolerance of potential antiinflammatory-analgesic agents have received increasing attention. Some of these factors are listed below.

Factors Influencing PG-Synthesis Inhibitors

1. Potency α Substrate Conc.
   Cofactor Conc.

2. Mode of inhibition - reversibility

3. Differential enzyme sensitivity vs. tissue origin
   synovium, platelet, etc.

4. Pharmacokinetics: Tissue distribution
   Duration of action

5. Spectrum of action vs. other arachidonic acid metabolites, oxidant radicals.

As the in vivo actions of prostaglandin synthetase inhibitors can no longer be compared or predicted solely on the basis of their relative potency in vitro, considerable mechanistic and pharmacodynamic studies are often devoted to the optimization of intrinsic drug activities, to improve potency and/or selectivity in vivo. A few discernable structure-activity relationships derived from these investigations are illustrated below.

2. IRREVERSIBLE AND REVERSIBLE CYCLOOXYGENASE INHIBITION

The facile and irreversible acetylation of cyclooxygenase, especially the platelet enzyme, by aspirin is well recognized (4). The high susceptibility of platelets underscores platelet dysfunction and bleeding tendency in antiarthritic therapy with aspirin. On the other hand, very low doses of aspirin, which preferentially inhibits platelet thromboxane synthetase

without affecting vascular prostacyclin synthetase, offers an interesting
approach to antithrombotic therapy (5).

The acetylation of the ε-amino group of a lysyl residue in cyclooxygenase is not solely determined by the chemical reactivity of the aromatic
acetate group. The stereochemical orientation of the inhibitor on the enzyme is also important. The requirement for specific binding in aspirin-
acetylation is evidenced by the higher rate of acetylation of cyclooxygenase
over serum albumin, and by the partial protection of cyclooxygenase against
aspirin inactivation by pretreatment with indomethacin or diflunisal (6).

The contour of a possible binding site for indomethacin and related
compounds on cyclooxygenase has been proposed recently on the basis of X-
ray coordinates of inhibitors and computer estimation of the probable con-
formation of the substrate arachidonic acid (7). It is composed of a hydrophobic pocket and a carboxyl binding site and generally accommodates many
aryl acidic cyclooxygenase inhibitors. However, except the carboxyl group

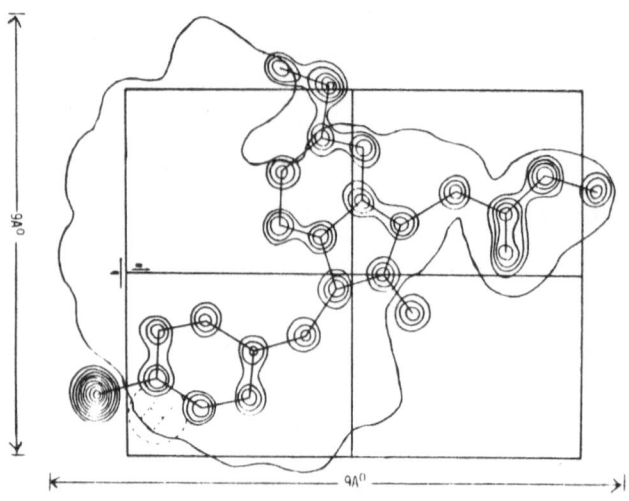

The superimposition of the X-ray projection of a sulindac analog
over the hypothetical binding site on cyclooxygenase.

at the anionic site, the precise orientation of the hydrophobic moiety in
different compounds are not always clear. In view of the partial but not
total protection of the enzyme provided by indomethacin and diflunisal, it
seems probable that the binding sites for these compounds are overlapping
but not identical with the binding site for aspirin. It is of special interest to note that the O-acetyl derivative of diflunisal, which may be
viewed as the 5-(2,4-difluorophenyl) derivative of aspirin,is incapable of
inactivating cyclooxygenase in vitro (8). Presumably the hydrophobic binding of the difluorophenyl moiety has reoriented the O-acetyl group in the
"aspirin portion" away from the lysyl ε-amino group. The benzoyl group in
indomethacin analogs is also chemically susceptible to nucleophilic cleavage.

Yet no significant transfer of a ^{3}H-labeled acyl group to cyclooxygenase was detected (9). This observation suggests that the carbonyl linkage in indomethacin is probably beyond the reach of the lysyl amino group in cyclooxygenase.

Schematic illustration of different, but overlapping, binding sites on the cyclooxygenase for aspirin, indomethacin and diflunisal acetate.

3. GASTROPROTECTIVE ACTIONS

Biologically, the competitive interaction of some NSAIDS at their overlapping sites on cyclooxygenase may be involved in the interesting gastroprotective action of NSAID combinations. Various pharmacological agents, e.g. carbenoxolone, antihistamines, etc. have been found to inhibit the gastric irritation induced by potent NSAIDS, e.g. indomethacin and phenylbutazone. More recently nonacidic and acidic NSAIDS, e.g. SL-573, a quinazolinone derivative (10), sodium salicylate (11), diflunisal and others, were reported to exert a similar gastroprotective action when given in combination with indomethacin in animal models. Competitive blockade of the binding

SL-573

of a potent inhibitor (indomethacin) to cyclooxygenase by a weaker inhibitor (SL-573) was suggested as a possible mechanism (10). The structure-activity relationship of gastroprotective agents and other biochemical considerations, e.g. protection vs. oxidant radical induced cyclooxygenase destruction, or alteration of the levels of different prostaglandins in target tissues remain to be clarified. The potential clinical application of these combinations is obvious.

4. DURATION OF ACTION

The overall drug effect is a function of intrinsic potency and the area under the curve of concentration vs. duration. Most NSAIDS, aspirin, indomethacin and aryl propionics, with serum half-life of 2-3 hrs., are generally given t.i.d. A longer acting prostaglandin synthesis inhibitor may possess advantages in terms of smaller and fewer dosage daily, and better patient compliance. Among factors affecting the pharmacodynamics and duration of action, enterohepatic recirculation and strong protein binding are common to many NSAIDS. Some, like naproxen, diflunisal and sulindac have longer serum half-life and are used in a b.i.d. schedule. The long half-life of sulindac sulfide (16.4 hrs) is sustained by its pharmacodynamics described below. The very long half-life (45 hrs) of piroxicam has been attributed to its chemical structure. The enolic form of piroxicam assumes two metabolically stable tautomers and, unlike antiinflammatory carboxylic acids, is not readily converted to glucuronide conjugate, etc. (12). Piroxicam sets an example of once a day therapy in arthritis.

5. IRREVERSIBLE AND REVERSIBLE PRODRUGS

Next, one may note a concept of reversible prodrugs. Prodrug is usually defined as an inactive substance which is metabolized to its active species in vivo. The metabolic activation processes, such as the hydrolysis of benorylate or an indomethacin ester and the oxidative degradation of a ketobutyric acid side-chain in fenbufen to give the more potent biphenylyl acetic acid (13), are irreversible. Similar oxidative activation probably takes place in the metabolism of furoprofen and bucloxic acid to generate more active species in vivo. Usually, after the initial phase of absorption, distribution and activation, the systemic pharmacokinetics of an irreversible prodrug is essentially similar to that of the active drug itself.

Irreversible Degradation of Prodrugs

Hydrolytic	Benorylate, Indomethacin ester and amide
Reductive	Imuran
Oxidative	Fenbufen

In contrast, the reduction of sulindac, a sulfoxide, to its active sulfide metabolite is reversible (14). A steady equilibrium, as measured by
serum concentration of metabolites, is quickly established in an hour or so.
However, the tissue concentration in different parts of the body varies according to the local enzymatic redox capacity and other distribution characteristics.

Reversible Activation of Prodrugs

Sulindac (sulfoxide)   **Sulfide Metabolite**

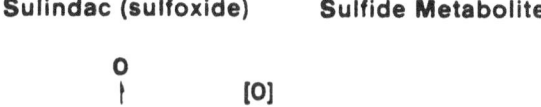

Systemic pharmacodynamics

function of tissue redox capacity
distribution characteristics

A. Reduced G.I. irritation

                                        O
                                        ↑
            Oral administration   [S]
                                              O
                                          ↑
        Enterohepatic recirculation   [S] >> [S]

B. Less effect on renal blood flow
                                            O
                                        ↑
                    local [S] vs. [S]

C. Antiinflammatory Efficacy

                                   O
$$\frac{[\text{Tissue}]}{[\text{Plasma}]} \quad [S] \;>>\; \overset{\uparrow}{[S]}$$

Based on extensive animal data and some clinical observations we feel
that the initial oral administration of the inactive sulfoxide and the pre-
ponderance of sulfoxide in enterohepatic recirculation minimize the exposure
of gastrointestinal tract to active drug and contribute to improved G.I.
tolerance. A preliminary clinical study indicated that sulindac seems to
produce less disturbance of renal blood flow than other NSAIDS (15), probably
due to more favorable sulfoxide distribution. On the other hand, tendency

of the active sulfide to accumulate in the inflammed tissues favors antiinflammatory efficacy of this reversible prodrug.

Such a complex but overall favorable pharmacodynamics of sulindac mainly results from the reversible conversion to its active sulfide. Interestingly, the same chemical reactivity of the sulfide group is responsible for the
oxidant radical scavenging effect (16). As the thio ether group often serves
as an effective halogen-equivalent in medicinal chemical studies, it may well
bring the reversible prodrug characteristics and oxidant radical scavenging
effect into other pharmacological agents. The well-known uricosuric-antiplate-
let agent, sulfinpyrazone, may be a hitherto unrecognized example. Indeed, we

Sulfinpyrazone   Sulfide Metabolite

have found that the sulfide analog, which is probably in equilibrium with
sulfinpyrazone in vivo, is much more potent as a cyclooxygenase and platelet
aggregation inhibitor and an oxidant radical scavenger than sulfinpyrazone itself in vitro. It would be of interest to see the incorporation of similar
sulfide substituents into antiinflammatory-analgesic and other pharmacological structures.

6. METABOLIC INACTIVATION OF TOPICAL ANTIINFLAMMATORY AGENTS

Prostaglandin synthesis inhibitors which are rapidly inactivated in vivo
do not possess systemic antiinflammatory efficacy and side-effects but may
still retain topical or local activities. For example, a group of non-acidic
cyclooxygenase inhibitors, 2-substituted phenyl [5,4-b] and [4,5-b] oxazolo-
pyridines have shown such selective actions. Among a large number of compounds investigated some are active in the carrageenan-edema and adjuvant
arthritis assays at 10-15 mg/kg p.o. (17). Several others in this series,
however, are highly effective in the guinea pig U.V. erythema assay but are
rapidly inactivated in vivo and devoid of any systemic effects (18). This
"reverse prodrug" approach may be of special interest in topical or local
applications.

[4,5-b]   [5,4-b]

Antiinflammatory 2-phenyl oxazolo pyridines.

7. CONCLUSION

In summary, prostaglandin synthetase inhibitors are non-equivalent in many aspects. Mechanism of action and pharmacodynamic studies offer a possible approach to enhance the in vivo efficacy and/or selectivity of active structures. Some specific chemical features have been associated with different modes of cyclooxygenase inhibition, gastroprotective action, duration of action and reversible prodrug pharmacodynamics. In particular, the sulfide-sulfoxide equilibrium in vivo and the antioxidant effect of some sulfide groups may find applications in other medicinal chemical studies.

REFERENCES

1. J. R. Vane, Nature, 231, 232 (1971).
2. R. J. Flower, Pharmacol. Rev., 26, 33 (1974).
3. T. Y. Shen in Antiinflammatory Drugs, J. R. Vane and S. H. Ferreira, Eds., Springer-Verlag, New York, 1978, p. 323.
4. G. J. Roth, N. Stanford and P. W. Majerus, Proc. Natl. Acad. Sci., U.S.A. 72, 3073 (1975).
5. J. W. Burch, N. Stanford and P. W. Majerus, J. Clin. Invest., 61, 314 (1978).
6. P. W. Majerus and N. Stanford, Brit. J. Clin. Pharmacol., 4, (Suppl. 1), 15 (1977).
7. P. Gund and T. Y. Shen, J. Med. Chem., 20,1146 (1977).
8. P. W. Majerus, Private communication.
9. N. Stanford, G. J. Roth, T. Y. Shen and P. W. Majerus, Prostaglandins, 13, 669 (1977).
10. Y. Yanagi and T. Komatsu, Biochem. Pharmacol., 25, 937 (1976).
11. E. Ezer, E. Palosi, Gy. Hajos, B. Rosdy and L. Szporny, Agents and Actions, 9, 117 (1979).
12. E. H. Wiseman, Y. H. Chang and J. G. Lombardino, Arzneim. Forsch., 26, 1300 (1976).
13. R. L. Tolman, J. E. Birnbaum, F. S. Chiccarelli, J. Panagides and A. E. Sloboda, in Advances in Prostaglandin and Thromboxane Res., B. Samuelsson and R. Paoletti, Eds., Raven Press, New York, 1976, p. 133.
14. D. E. Duggan, K. F. Hooke, E. A. Risley, T. Y. Shen and C. G. Van Arman, J. Pharmacol. Exptl. Therap., 201, 8 (1977).
15. C. Patrono, Private communication.
16. R. W. Egan, P. H. Gale, W. J. A. Vandenheuvel and F. A. Kuehl, the following paper.
17. R. L. Clark, A. A. Pessolano, B. Witzel, T. Lanza, T. Y. Shen, C. G. Van Arman and E. A. Risley, J. Med. Chem., 21, 1158 (1978).
18. N. P. Jensen, et al., Unpublished results.

THE GUINEA-PIG ISOLATED ILEUM AS A MODEL FOR THE STUDY OF PROSTAGLANDINS INTERACTIONS WITH ANTIINFLAMMATORY DRUGS

J.P.FAMAEY, J.FONTAINE AND J.REUSE
Laboratory of Pharmacology, School of Medicine and Institute of
Pharmacy, University of Brussels, Brussels, Belgium

Most of the antirheumatic compounds interfere with Prostaglandins (PGs) production or function. These interferences lead generally to a decrease of PGs in the inflamed tissues as it is the case with aspirin -like drugs,antiinflammatory steroids and mepacrine. With other compounds like gold salts and D-penicillamine known as long-acting antirheumatic drugs an increase in the production of PGEs has been described which might be relevant for the treatment of chronic inflammation. A third effect might be an antagonistic effect like that observed with chloroquine on vascular smooth muscle (1).

Any simple model for the study of PGs should be a good one too for the study of antirheumatic compounds. This might be the case for the guinea-pig isolated ileum. This model has been extensively studied. Many data concerning the possible role of PGs in this smooth muscle were obtained by adding indomethacin or other aspirin-like drugs to the incubation bath as a tool for inhibiting the ileal PG-synthetase. However the added drugs' concentrations were sometimes large enough to allow other biochemical interpretations of the results (2). We decided thus to focus our attention on the interactions between various contractile agonists including the PGs themselves and several antirheumatic compounds in this simple peculiar model.

Our previous works in this field can be briefly summarized. The aspirin-like drugs and the antiinflammatory steroids inhibit any kind of contractile responses. The effect was more pronounced for aspirin-like drugs on responses to indirect agonists and to histamine. These ganglioplegic and antihistaminic properties were not observed for antiinflammatory steroids. Regardless to the agonist used PGs abolish these inhibitions (3,4,5).

We have observed what was also described previously by others that PGs are able to potentiate non specifically any kind of ileal contractions (5). This suggests that the reversal by PGs of inhibitions by antiinflammatory compounds might be merely related to the ability of PGs to non selectively improve smooth muscle contractility rather than to PG requirement for some specific agonist to exert its action as it was claimed for cholinergic agonists. The inhibition by antiinflam-

matory compounds should be also largely non selective related
perhaps to their well known effects on biological membranes.
          These conclusions were reinforced by two different
observations. First we have obtained similar inhibitions with
non antiinflammatory steroids like sex steroid hormones (6,7)
and mineralocorticosteroids (8). Secondly we observed a reversal
of all these inhibitions by non prostaglandinic compounds like
the polypeptides caerulein and physalaemin which were also
able to non selectively sensitize the ileal smooth muscle to
a large range of agonists (9).
          If a specific inhibitor of PG-synthesis(indomethacin)
would selectively inhibit contractions to acetylcholine and
other cholinergic agonists and if this inhibition would be
exclusively reversed by PG it might be concluded that PG production is required for observing cholinergic ileal contractions.
But what can be concluded from inhibition by oestrogens reversed
by caerulein except that unspecific inhibitions are abolished
by unspecific potentiating agents and that perhaps a series
of literature data obtained in this model by using antiinflammatory drugs should be reconsidered at the light of this.
          Moreover at the high concentrations used in most of
these experiments we were able to show an antagonistic effect
on PGs action on the ileum for both steroids, including sex
steroids, and non steroidal antiinflammatory drugs (10,11).
          It can be thus concluded that great precautions must
be taken in drawing conclusions from results obtained with
specific inhibitions of PG synthesis or production when used
at high concentrations.
          More positive results have been also obtained by
using this model. This was the case by using drugs known to
increase PG production in certain circumstances. Theoretically
by increasing productions of ileal PGs they should mimic the
potentiation observed with exogenously added PGs. This was
actually obtained with colchicine (12), with vinblastine (13)
and D-penicillamine (14). This was apparently also observed
with several other sulfhydryl agents as suggested by some of
our presently unpublished data. An inhibition of these increases by not too high concentrations of aspirin-like drugs
in some experiments might be related to effects on PGs. Whether
those are actually increased in the incubate should be only
demonstrated by selective dosages.
          Recently we extended our investigations to a whole
series of antimalarial compounds with the aim of finding differences between those with and those without antirheumatic
properties. We have obtained rather puzzling preliminary
results. We were unable to find any selective antagonism to
PGs actions in our preparation as it was observed for chloro-
quine (15), quinacrine and quinine in vascular smooth muscle
preparations. These antimalarials were merely non specific
inhibitors for all kinds of agonists. These inhibitions were
counteracted non specifically by PGs.
          Similar observations were made with chlorguanide

(Paludrine) which was used in the 1950 in France for treating some cases of rheumatoid arthritis, as well as with non anti-malarial biguanides such as the antidiabetic compounds phen-formine and metformine. It has been suggested however that biguanides would be able in certain preparations to stimulate the production of a PGE_1 like compound.

The most exciting preliminary data were obtained with amodiaquine and primaquine.

Amodiaquine is a 4-aminoquinoline and thus a chloro-quine congener which has been used in the treatment of rheuma-toid arthritis but was abandoned because of blood and hepatic toxicity.

This compound behaves in many aspects like PGs. It potentiates very nicely all kinds of ileal responses at low do-ses and reverses several types of inhibition. At higher doses it induces reproducible dose dependent contraction by acting directly on the muscle itself. These contractions were not abolished by tetrodotoxin but were sensitive to indomethacin as well as to the PG antagonist polyphloretin phosphate.

Primaquine on the other hand was an 8-aminoquinoline with very strong antimalarial properties but devoid of any antirheumatic properties.

It similarly potentiates ileal contractions at low doses and induces contractions at higher doses. These were only sensitive to H_1 antagonists such as mepyramine. This suggests a role for primaquine on histamine receptors.

Whether these observations on antimalarials are purely academic or related to pharmacological or toxicological effects including antirheumatic or even antimalarial effects remains a moot point for the moment.

In conclusion it seems that the guinea-pig isolated ileum would be a simple model on which antirheumatic drugs might be screened for confirming some of their pharmacological properties, questioning others and even discovering new ones which then should be allowed to be tested on more classical models of inflammation.

REFERENCES

(1) J.P.FAMAEY, Recent developments about non-steroidal anti-
     inflammatory drugs and their mode of action,*Gen.Pharmac.*,
     9, 155-162 (1978)
(2) S.EHRENPREIS, J.GREENBERG and S.BELMAN,Prostaglandins re-
     verse inhibition of electrically induced contractions of
     guinea-pig ileum by morphine, indomethacin and acetylsali-
     cylic acid,*Nature, New Biol.* 245, 280-282 (1973)
(3) J.P.FAMAEY,J.FONTAINE and J.REUSE, The inhibiting effect of
     morphine, chloroquine, non-steroidal and steroidal antiin-
     flammatory drugs on the electrically induced contractions
     of guinea-pig ileum smooth muscle and the reversing effects
     of prostaglandins, *Agents Actions*, 5, 354-358 (1975)
(4) J.P.FAMAEY, J.FONTAINE and J.REUSE, The effect of non-
     steroidal antiinflammatory drugs on cholinergic and
     histamine-induced contractions of guinea-pig isolated ileum,
     Br. J. Pharmac.,60, 165-171 (1977)
(5) J.P.FAMAEY, J.FONTAINE,I.SEAMAN and J.REUSE, The effects of
     various antiinflammatory steroids on contractions of
     guinea-pig isolated ileum to acetylcholine, histamine,
     nicotine, 5-hydroxytryptamine and electrical stimulations,
     Naunyn-Schmiedeberg's Arch. Pharmac.,in press (1979)
(6) I.SEAMAN, J.P.FAMAEY, J.FONTAINE and J.REUSE, Inhibitory
     effects of sexual steroid hormones on the responses of the
     guinea-pig isolated ileum to acetylcholine and histamine,
     Arch. Int. Pharmacodyn. Thér.,227, 233-237 (1977)
(7) I.SEAMAN, J.FONTAINE, J.P.FAMAEY and J.REUSE, The inhibitory
     effects of steroidal sex hormones on the responses of the
     guinea-pig isolated ileum to nicotine and serotonine,*Arch.
     Int. Pharmacodyn. Thér.*,230, 340-343 (1977)
(8) J.FONTAINE, I.SEAMAN, J.P.FAMAEY and J.REUSE, The inhibitory
     effects of two mineralocorticoids (aldosterone and desoxy-
     corticosterone) on the responses of the guinea-pig isolated
     ileum to several agonists, *Arch. Int. Pharmacodyn. Thér.*,
     232, 336-338 (1978)
(9) J.P.FAMAEY, J.FONTAINE and J.REUSE, Interactions of non-
     steroidal antiinflammatory drugs with substance P-like
     and gastrointestinal hormones-like polypeptides, *in
     "Perspectives in inflammation : Future trends and develop-
     ment" Eds D.A. Willoughby, J.P.Giroud and G.P. Velo, M.T.P.
     Press Limited*, pp 347-352 (1977)
(10) J.P.FAMAEY, J.FONTAINE and J.REUSE, Effect of high concen-
     trations of non-steroidal and steroidal antiinflammatory
     drugs on prostaglandin induced contractions of the guinea-
     pig isolated ileum, *Prostaglandins*, 13, 107-114 (1977)
(11) I.SEAMAN, J.FONTAINE, J.P.FAMAEY and J.REUSE, An analysis
     of the inhibitory effects and of possible prostaglandins
     antagonism of sex steroid hormones in the guinea-pig ileum,
     J.Pharm. Pharmac.,30, 525-526 (1978)
(12) J.P.FAMAEY, J. FONTAINE and J.REUSE, Smooth muscle sensiti-
     zation induced by colchicine: is it an in vitro property

of antitubulin agents ?,*Agents Actions*, 7, 305-309(1977)

(13) J.P.FAMAEY,J. FONTAINE and J.REUSE, Smooth muscle
sensitization induced by vinblastine, *Agents Actions*,
6, 724-727 (1976)

(14) J.P.FAMAEY, J.FONTAINE and J.REUSE, The effects of
D-penicillamine on ileal smooth muscle and their
possible relationships with prostaglandins,*in "Penicil-
lamine research in rheumatoid disease"* Ed. E. Munthe,
pp 50-58 *Fabritius and Sønner, Oslo* (1976)

(15) J.P.FAMAEY, J.FONTAINE and J.REUSE, An analysis of the
inhibitory effects and of possible prostaglandins antagonism of chloroquine in the guinea-pig isolated ileum
J. *Pharm. Pharmac.*, 29, 761-762 (1977)

Chapter Five

PROSTAGLANDINS AND SIDE-EFFECTS OF ANTI-INFLAMMATORY
DRUGS

PROSTAGLANDINS AND THE DEVELOPMENT OF GASTRIC MUCOSAL DAMAGE BY ANTI-INFLAMMATORY DRUGS

K.D. Rainsford
Biochemistry Department, University of Tasmania, Medical School,
G.P.O. Box 252 C, Hobart, Tasmania, Australia 7001

Inhibition of prostaglandin (PG) synthesis and release has been
suggested as a major factor in the development of gastro-intestinal ulceration and haemorrhage induced by the anti-inflammatory drugs (1-3). Moreover, alterations in mucosal PG
production have been implicated in the aetiology of gastric
ulcer diseases (e.g. resulting from exposure to stress states)
and inflammatory conditions of the gastro-intestinal tract,
e.g. ulcerative colitis (4,5). The sheer volume of literature
implicating prostaglandins in the development of experiment-
ally-induced gastric ulceration in laboratory animals is most
impressive (2,3). Experiments of the kind showing the protective effects of E-type or other prostaglandins on gastric or
intestinal damage included by non-steroid anti-inflammatory
(NSAI) drugs or other agents is also most striking. Yet on analysis some of this and other experimental evidence must be critically assessed. While it is true that current evidence suggests that effects on prostaglandin synthesis do seem to be important in the development of gastric mucosal damage induced
by NSAI drugs, the problem at present is to know at precisely
what stage these effects are important. This is especially so
as various other physiological and biochemical effects of these
drugs (e.g. inhibition of ATP production, intermediary metabolism, mucus biosynthesis, K-ATPase, membrane damage, cytologi-
cal or cytotoxic effects) all appear to be involved in the
development of gastric mucosal damage (6-10).

First, however, it is important to reiterate two important factors which are fundamental to understanding the development of
NSAI drug-induced gastric damage (6), namely:

(1) The mechanism of gastric mucosal damage has a multifacto-
     rial basis.

(2) Systemic as well as local factors are both important. The
     relative contribution of these factors is dependant on the
     time and dosage of drug and thus the concentration of drug

following absorption from the gastric lumen or from the
uptake into mucosal tissue of the drug or its metabolites
in circulation.

Systemic manifestations may not only result from the presence
of the drug within the mucosa but may also be consequent upon
actions on other organ systems, e.g. CNS control of vagal acti-
vitiy (and hence acid secretion), physiological or pathological
variations in drug metabolism by the liver etc. Actual amounts
of the drug or its metabolites absorbed by the mucosa from the
systemic circulation will depend on the amount of drug bound to
circulating plasma proteins. The situation concerning pro-drugs,
(e.g. sulindac, fenbufen, meseclazone) which are metabolized to
active products is more complex since the activities of enzymes
involved in drug metabolism will be an important factor in determining the contribution of the drug or its metabolic product
which is effective as an inhibitor of prostaglandin production
or any other biochemical process of significance in the pathogenesis of gastric mucosal damage.

These are particularly important factors in the case of damage
induced by aspirin - one of the drugs principally implicated in
gastric ulceration and haemorrhage in the population (6). Appreciable hydrolysis of aspirin occurs in both the gastric mucosa
and blood due to the activities of aspirin esterases, as well
as through spontaneous hydrolysis (11-14). The amount of aspirin, compared with salicylate, present in the mucosa and in the
systemic circulation will largely depend on the activities of aspirin esterases. This is of particularly significance since aspirin is not only more ulcerogenic than its immediate metabolite,
salicylate (15) but it has different metabolic effects: the most
significant in the context of the present discussion being that
aspirin a more potent inhibitor of prostaglandin synthesis than
salicylate (16).

Finally, when considering the propensitiy of different NSAI
drugs to cause gastric ulceration it is important to remember
that oral administration of these drugs at therapeutic dose ranges to (unstressed) experimental animals, with the possible exception of potent drugs e.g. indomethacin, rarely results in
gastric ulceration per se (i.e. perforation of the mucosa) but
only induces superficial lesions. Many other factors may contribute to the pathogenesis of ulceration including such factors as
stress states, tablet preparations etc. (14, 17). It is against
this background of complex factors involved in the pathogenesis
of gastric mucosal damage induced by NSAI drugs that role of
prostaglandins must be considered.

1. ACTIONS OF PROSTAGLANDINS AND RELATIONSHIP TO ANTI-ULCER
   ACTIVITIES.

Extensive studies have been performed showing the protective
effects of exogenously administered prostaglandins (PG's), including both the natural and long-acting synthetic PG's (see
also reviews in extenso in refs. 2 and 4). In summary, these
studies have shown that:

(1) A wide variety of PG's will, when given orally or par-
    enterally, inhibit the formation of gastric lesions
    induced not only by NSAI drugs but a wide variety of
    noxious or stress-inducing agents (2,3,4,14,18). The
    effects of the PG's on inhibiting the development of
    gastric (fundic) lesions by NSAI drugs is evident re-
    gardless of whether these drugs are given orally or
    parenterally. Intestinal lesions induced by drugs such
    as indomethacin are likewise inhibited by oral or par-
    enteral doses of PG's (21) although the mechanism of
    inhibition by PG's is probably somewhat different to
    that in the stomach (2).

(2) Inhibitory effects of PG's on lesion formation in the
    fundic mucosa has been related to:

    a) Reduction in acid output which may be an indirect
       effect related to vascular effects of PG's in the
       stomach (2,3,14,18,19).

    b) Enhancement of blood flow (14,18,20) and blood
       content (21) (the latter possibly reflecting the
       generalized vasodilator actions particularly of
       PGE's) together with reduced peripheral resistance
       and gastric arterial pressure (20). Tissue water
       content, also increases markedly (22).

    c) Protection against mast cell degranulation (23)
       which may be of particular significance since the
       histamine content of the gastric mucosa increases
       after administration of aspirin and other NSAI-
       drugs (6). Also mast cell degranulation occurs in
       the mucosa after exposure to stress (6). The H_2-
       receptor antagonists (e.g. metiamide, cimetidine)
       are most effective in reducing most types of
       stress or drug-induced ulceration (3,14). This is
       probably a reflection of the effects of histmine
       in gastric ulcerogenesis.

    d) An apparent "cytoprotective" effect on mucosal
       cells independent of effects on acid secretion (2,
       24,25). This cytoprotective effect could be mani-

fest through discharge of mucus and a watery like
fluid from surface mucosal cells together with enhanced water content of the fundic mucosa (22) -
see Fig. 1. The cyto-protective effect may be consequence of administering such potent and well
known irritants as the PG's so leading to the same
effects on the gastric mucosa as other chemical
irritants (26). Whether or not <u>endogenous</u> PG's
have natural cytoprotective actions is still unre-
solved.

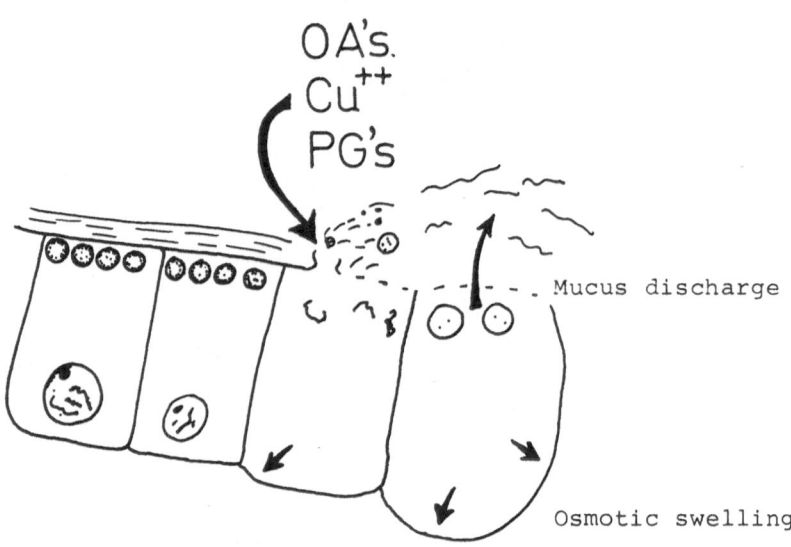

Fig.1: Possible actions of chemical irritants in promoting
mucus discharge from the gastric mucous cells - an effect that
could account for the "cytoprotective" actions of these
agents. Organic acids (e.g. prostaglandins, weak acids including
aspirin,salicylic acid etc.) or Cu^{++} ions (see ref. 26) may
cause changes in membrane permeability of surface mucous cells
so leading to increased swelling from osmotic effects and
subsequent discharge of mucus-containing globules present in
mucous cells. Such mucus discharge may, by a positive outward
flow, serve to reduce the interaction of ulcerogenic drugs
with the mucosa when these drugs are administered orally. Also,
the mucus discharge may mask the appearance, or even development
of, haemorrhagic events in the mucosa. Protection by prostaglandins
against damage by NSAI drugs given parenterally may also be
due to permeability changes (induced by PG's) leading to enhanced
osmotic swelling and "positive resistence" against drug uptake.
The organic acids (including PG's) or Cu^{++}ions may also elicit
endogenous prostaglandin release following mobilization of
phospholipids so contributing to osmotic changes in the mucosa.

It must, therefore, be concluded that exogenous administration of what appear to be large doses of PG's can only be regarded as producing in sensu stricto pharmacologic effects. Any relationship to physiologic role of alterations in the endogenous concentrations of PG's by drugs of other ulcerogenic agents from this kind of evidence must be subject to these reservations.

2. ACTIONS OF ENDOGENOUS PROSTAGLANDINS.

The endogenous PG's in the stomach are principally 6-keto PGF_1 (from degradation of PGI_2) and PGE_2 or its degradation products (27-30). It is of interest that PGI_2 (prostacyclin) is a more potent inhibitor of acid secretion than either its breakdown product, 6-keto PGF_1, or PGE_2 (18). However, PGI_2 is only equipotent with PGE_2 in inhibiting indomethacin-induced gastric ulceration in rats (18). These differences may be related to either direct pharmacological effects or differences in the degradation rates of these PG's.

To identify a common mechanism or site for action of PG's and NSAI drugs on the gastric mucosa would seem difficult in view of the multiplicity of actions of these drugs/compounds. However, in relation to acid secretion it is possible that effects of PG's on mucosal cyclic AMP concentrations may, in part, explain the actions of both these substances (31,32). This is especially so since intracellular cyclic AMP has been linked with the regulation of acid secretion (33-35). Aspirin has been shown to increase the concentrations of cyclic AMP in the rat gastric mucosa in vivo (31,32). High concentrations (6.6 mM) of aspirin and salicylate increased the cyclic AMP content of minced mucosa in vitro (36). While these effects require confirmation at lower drug concentrations it is noteworthy that prostaglandin E_1 (10^{-5}M) reversed the levels of cyclic AMP elevated by the salicylates. This effect was also observed with metiamide - the H_2-receptor antagonist with anti-ulcer action (36). Both PGE_2 and, at higher concentrations, PGI_2 inhibit the accumulation of ^{14}C-labelled aminopyrine (used as an index of acid secretion in vitro in isolated canine parietal cells (37)). This has been related to effects of PG's in reversing the cyclic AMP levels elevated by histamine (37). While these results appear attractive in the sense of relating effects of NSAI drugs and PG's to cyclic nucleotide production there is one report that prostaglandins E_2, A_2 and their methylated analogues increase adenyl cyclase activity in the human gastric mucosa (38). Since aspirin and other NSAI drugs inhibit the PG-stimulated adenyl cyclase in human astrocytoma cells in culture (39) it remains a possibility that similar antagonism of PG-regulation of acid secretion in the stomach could occur. Certainly, the situation is probably quite complex and it still remains for the metabolic aspects of gastric proton production (40,41) to be evaluated in the light of drug effects on both ATP and cyclic nucleotide production.

Table 1: EFFECTS OF CO-ADMINISTRATION OF ARACHIDONATE OR PG
ENDOPEROXIDE ANALOGUE,ON ASPIRIN, OR INDOMETHACIN-
INDUCED GASTRIC LESIONS IN STRESSED RATS

Expt. No.	Treatment	Number of Lesions (mean ± S.E.)	Lesion
1.	Aspirin (150 mg/kg p.o.)alone	27.3 ± 2.3	39.6
	- with cholesterol arachido- nate (100 mg/kg p.o.)	39.7 ± 1.7	51.7
2.	Indomethacin (10 mg/kg p.o.) alone	54.7 ± 7.4	65.7
	- with arachidonic acid (100 mg/kg p.o.)	62.5 ± 9.2	73.0
	- with cholesterol arachido- nate (100 mg/kg p.o.)	39.7 ± 1.7	51.7
3.	Aspirin (100 mg/kg p.o.) alone	34.0 ± 5.5	47.3
	- with U44069 (1 mg/kg i.p.)	19.3 ± 2.7	31.0
4.	Aspirin (100 mg/kg p.o.) alone	23.8 ± 3.0	37.3
	- with U44069 (1 mg/kg p.o.)	23.0 ± 8.4	36.5
	- with PGE_2 (5 mg/kg p.o.)	5.0 ± 2.2*	13.8
5.	Indomethacin (10 mg/kg p.o.) alone	49.7 ±12.8	60.7
	- with U44069 (1 mg/kg i.p.)	24.3 ± 2.9	35.3

U44069 = (15S) -hydroxy-9, 11-(epoxymethano)prosta 5Z,
13E-dienoic acid.
Procedures as in ref. 14 with lesions numbers and severity
recorded in groups 4-6 fasted (24 hrs) rats 2 hrs after drug
administration and concomitant exposure to cold (-15°,
35 mins) stress conditions. PGE_2 was administered to one
group of rats in these series as a positive control to relate to the previous studies (14).

* Statistically significant reduction c.f. aspirin alone
  (P< 0.05, 't'-test).

3. EFFECTS OF PROSTAGLANDIN PRECURSORS ON GASTRIC ULCERATION BY
   ANTI-INFLAMMATORY DRUGS.

Recently, it was found that co-administration of even high doses
(35 mg/kg) the PG precursor, arachidonic acid, failed to inhibit
the gastric damage induced by aspirin in a sensitive and specific model for determining gastric ulcerogenic activity - the
stressed rat (14). Also, as shown in Table 1, co-administered
cholesterol arachidonate likewise failed to inhibit gastric damage in stressed rats induced by either aspirin or indomethacin.
The ester was employed in these studies to obviate any irritant
effects which might be due to administration of the acid itself.
The sodium salt of arachidonate was also ineffective in reducing
the gastric damage induced by aspirin (data not shown). These
results raise the question as to whether or not the endoperoxides derived from arachidonic acid i.e. PGG_2 and PGH_2 may be of
any importance in the development of gastric damage. It could be
argued that the blockade of endoperoxide (and PG production) by
aspirin or indomethacin could be so effective as to prevent any
PG's being generated in the gastric mucosa. For this reason it
was decided to examine the effects of co-administering a stable
synthetic endoperoxide derivative U44069 (Upjohn). As shown in
Table 1 this derivative had no effect when given orally and was
slightly effective when given parenterally in reducing the gastric mucosal damage induced by aspirin or indomethacin. These
results suggest that endoperoxides may only be of slight significance in protecting the mucosa against NSAI drugs induced damage. However, these stable endoperoxides may induce changes in
PG metabolism so that these results can only serve as indicating
potential role of endoperoxides.

Another approach to understanding the role of PGG_2 or PGH_2 in
drug-induced ulceration is to employ drugs that manipulate or
change the levels of endoperoxides in cells. Such a strategy
could include using drugs which act to scavenge free radicals generated on conversion of PGG_2 to PGH_2, in the peroxidase reaction
(42,43). The effect of these drugs on arachidonate metabolism
would be to increase the production of PGH_2 and subsequent PG metabolites (42,43).

Kuehl and co-workers have suggested (42,43) that free oxygen
radicals (O) produced as a consequence of the peroxidase reaction can be scavenged by phenolic drugs such as MK-447 (2-
aminoethyl, 4 t-butyl, 6-iodo-phenol), salicylate or diflunisal (2,4-difluoro-5-phenyl-salicylic acid). Free-radical sca-
vengers would also be expected to over-ride the inhibition by
NSAI drugs of the cyclo-oxygenase reactions (i.e. involving the
conversion of arachidonate to PGH_2). Interestingly, Ezer and co-
workers (44) have shown that salicylate attenuates the irritant
effects of indomethacin and other NSAI drugs on the gastric and

Table 2: EFFECTS OF CO-ADMINISTERING PHENOLIC COMPOUNDS ON
         GASTRIC DAMAGE INDUCED BY INDOMETHACIN IN RATS

Drug treatment (dose, mg/kg)	Number of Lesions (mean $\pm$ S.E.)	Lesion Index
1. Indomethacin (0.2)	3.0 $\pm$ 0.9	11.5
- with MK-447 (1.2)	1.8 $\pm$ 1.0	7.3
2. Indomethacin (10)	48.0 $\pm$ 10.4	59.3
- with MK-447 (60)*	0 **	0
3. Indomethacin (2)	3.3 $\pm$ 1.7	11.6
- with Na-salicylate (10)	4.3 $\pm$ 2.0	13.0
- with Na-salicylate (100)	0.5 $\pm$ 0.1	10.5
4. Indomethacin (10)	33.0 $\pm$ 7.4	44.0
- with Na-salicylate (100)	29.7 $\pm$ 3.5	42.4
5. Indomethacin (10)	49.7 $\pm$ 12.6	60.7
- with paracetamol (50)	61.8 $\pm$ 8.3	72.8

*   Mucus effusion evident at 60 and 120 mg/kg doses of mixture.

N = 4-5 per group. Procedures as described in ref. 14 - see
    also Table 1. All doses p.o. in quantities given in
    brackets.

** Significant decrease in number of lesions ('t'-test, $P < 0.05$).

intestinal mucosa (in unstressed rats). These authors suggested
that the effect of salicylate might be to act as a less effective agent in "unbalancing" the prostaglandin "equilibrum"
affected by potent inhibitors such as aspirin. The free-radical
scavenging effects of salicylate could be one plausible mechanism for correcting the "inbalance" as suggested by these authors.

In the stress-sensitized gastric ulcer assay, which we have employed, both MK-447 and diflunisal were found to inhibit the
ulcerogenic effects of aspirin and indomethacin with salicylate
being somewhat less effective than either of these drugs (Table
2 and ref. 45). Paracetamol was totally ineffective in preventing indomethacin induced gastric ulceration in this assay.

There is, however, one further action which has not been considered this is that drugs with specific irritant actions, such as
salicylate will induce an appreciable amount of mucus effusion or
discharge from mucus cells (15). In the present work potent mucus
discharge was noticed with MK-447. This effect could arise from
either the influence of the drug in stimulating PG production in
vivo to such levels as to cause an endogenous type of mucus discharge or from the direct irritant actions of these phenolic compounds on the gastric mucosa as observed other irritants (22).
The lack of any protective effects of paracetamol might be due to
this drug being less effective either as a free radical scavenger
in vivo (quantitatively speaking) or in inducing the mucus effusion response exhibited by the other phenolic compounds.

4. RELATIONSHIP BETWEEN INHIBITION OF PROSTAGLANDIN BIOSYNTHESIS
   AND GASTRIC ULCERATION BY NSAI DRUGS.

Several authors have attempted to correlate inhibition effects
of NSAI drugs on PG synthesis in vitro with their propensity to
induce gastric damage (46,47). In one such study (47) a correlation was claimed to exist between PG inhibitory potency calculated on a millimolar concentration basis with an ED_{50} dose required for gastro-intestinal bleeding on a mg for body weight
basis. For consistency the doses of drugs for the gastro-intestinal bleeding studies should have been calculated a millimoles
per kg. body weight basis. There is a technical aspect that
gastro-intestinal bleeding measured by the method used by these
authors may be inaccurate (6,49). Also, it was notable that the
correlation between inhibitory potency of NSAI drugs on PG production and gastro-intestinal bleeding rested entirely on a
single point (i.e. aspirin).

In recent studies where the structure of individual groups of
NSAI drugs was compared with their ulcerogenic activity it was
apparent that physio-chemical parameters, such as lipid solubi-

Table 3: COMPARISON OF GASTRIC ULCEROGENIC ACTIVITY OF ANTI-
         INFLAMMATORY DRUGS WITH THEIR PROSTAGLANDIN "ANTI-
         SYNTHETASE" ACTIVITY

Drug	Gastric ulcer* ED_{10} mmol/kg	Gut PGE** ED_{50} mM
Aspirin	0.018	3.30
Indomethacin	0.014	0.0084
Naproxen	0.0006	0.0065
Phenylbutazone	0.122	0.032
Diclofenac	0.017	0.0003
Ibuprofen	0.070	0.029

Correlation analysis Hansch-type equation:

$$Log \frac{1}{ED_{10}} = 0.471 \ (\pm 0.797)(Log\ P)^2 - 1.734 \ (\pm 1.105) Log\ P - 0.678$$

$$(\pm 0.344)\ PG\ ED_{50} + 1.314 \ (\pm 0.509)$$

$$Correlation\ coeff.\ R = 0.691\ (P < 0.05)$$

*   Assayed according to the procedure in ref. 14. See also
     table 1. ED_{10} is the dose required to produce 10 lesions
     obtained from dose-response curves (48).

** Data from ref. 47.

lity (expressed as the log of the partition coefficient, i.e.
log P) or pKa are important in determining the ulcerogenic activity of these drugs (48). Absorption of these drugs in the stomach and other factors possibly relating to their local irri-
tant/ulcerogenic actions in the development of gastric mucosal
damage likewise depends on these physico-chemical parameters.
Using the conventional Hansch analysis (49) no direct correlation was observed between ulcerogenic activity and physico-chemical properties across a wide range of acidic NSAI drugs although the previous studies (48) had shown that these parameters
were related within individual structural types (e.g. salicylates). Other factors relating to the biochemical actions of specific chemical moieties of different NSAI drugs, e.g. potency in
inhibiting PG synthesis, could be implicated with physico-chemical properties of these drugs in determining their ulcerogenic
actions. The results in Tables 3 and 4 show that a correlation
does exist of both lipid solubility (log P) and prostaglandin
inhibition data with ulcerogenic activity. Such correlation held
regardless of whether the data on effects on PG synthesis was
derived from studies on gut or bovine seminal vesicle enzymes.
It is tempting to speculate from these experiments in terms of a
model system in which ulcerogenic action of NSAI drug could depend on (1) absorption of the drug into mucosal cells (dependent
on log P and pKa), and (2) steric and physicochemical factors
(including lipid solubility and electronic factors) which would
determine in turn the likelihood of interaction of the drug with
the PG "synthetase" enzyme complexes.

Physical disruption of membranes leading to permeability changes in the gastric mucosa by irritant NSAI drugs (6) following
absorption or interaction of the drugs with the lipid components
in membranes could also be considered as part of complex biochemical mechanism in this particular model. However, it is necessary to caution on extrapolation of effects of drugs on in
vitro in such systems as the PG synthesis assays; especially
since there is controversy over the role of co-factors in the enzyme assays which are employed in these studies (16). What these
studies may provide is a possible working model for establishing
the relationship of biochemical actions of drugs, not only as
inhibitors of PG synthesis, but other effects e.g. uncoupling of
oxidative phosphorylation (6).

5. CONCLUSIONS.

It appears that some correlation may exist between effects of
NSAI drugs on PG metabolism and their ulcerogenic activity. It
is clear from the studies presented and discussed here that
there are many inherant difficulties in experiments designed to
establish exactly in what way effects on PG metabolism influence
the development of gastric mucosal damage induced by NSAI drugs.

Table 4: COMPARISON OF GASTRIC ULCEROGENIC ACTIVITY OF ANTI-
         INFLAMMATORY DRUGS WITH PROSTAGLANDIN "ANTI-SYNTHETASE"
         ACTIVITY

Drug	Gastric ulcer* ED_{10} mmol/kg	B.S.V. PGE_2** ED_{50} mM
Aspirin	0.018	23.2
Diclofenac	0.017	0.0046
Fenoprofen	0.040	0.062
Flufenamic acid	0.197	0.006
Ibuprofen	0.070	0.120
Indomethacin	0.0136	0.0105
Mefenamic acid	0.71	0.004
Naproxen	0.0006	0.032
Phenylbutazone	0.122	0.204
Tolmetin	0.017	0.0117

Correlation analysis Hansch type equation:

$$Log \frac{1}{ED_{10}} = -0.364(\pm0.239)(Log\ P)^2 - 0.174(\pm0.453)Log\ P + 0.255(\pm0.212)PG\ ED_{50} + 2.533(\pm0.538)$$

$$r = 0.732,\ P < 0.05$$

* Procedures for assay of gastric ulcerogenic activity as in
  ref. 14. ED_{10} is the dose required to produce 10 lesions.

** Data from ref. 50 using bovine seminal vesicle microsomal
   preparation as source of enzymes for PG synthesis in vitro.

Establishing a correlation is one thing but defining the basis
of this correlation is another. The large number of studies
where exogenous application of PG's has been employed are insufficient evidence alone (vide supra). This aspect has been
pointed out by Needleman (49) to apply as well in other systems
where the role PG's has been studied.

Acknowledgements:

My thanks to Messrs. D. Jacobs, M. Plaister and Miss D. Clennent
for help in maintenance and help with the animals.

REFERENCES

(1) J.R. VANE. Inhibition of Prostaglandin Synthesis as a Me-
     chanism of Action of Aspirin-like Drugs. Nature New Biol.
     231, 232-235 (1971).

(2) A. ROBERT. Antisecretory, Antiulcer, Cytoprotective and
     Diarrhoegenic Properties of Prostaglandins. In: Advances
     in Prostaglandin and Thromboxane Research 2, 507-520 (1976).

(3) B.J.R. WHITTLE. Relationship between the Prevention of Rat
     Gastric Erosions and the Inhibition of Acid Secretion by
     Prostaglandins. Eur. J. Pharmacol. 40, 233-239 (1976).

(4) A. BENNETT. Prostaglandins as Factors in Diseases of the
     Alimentary Tract. In: Advances in Prostaglandin and Thrombo-
     xane Research 2, 547-555 (1976).

(5) D.W. HARRIS, P.R. SMITH and C.S.H. SWAN. Determination of
     Prostaglandin Synthetase Activity in Rectal Biopsy Material
     and its Significance in Colonic Disease. Gut 19, 875-877
     (1978).

(6) K.D. RAINSFORD. The Biochemical Pathology of Aspirin-induced
     Gastric Damage. Agents and Actions 5, 326-344 (1975).

(7) T.G. JORGENSEN, U.S. WEIS-FOGH and H.P. OLESEN. The Influ-
     ence of Acetylsalicylic Acid (Aspirin) on Gastric Mucosal
     Content of Energy-Rich Phosphate Bonds. Scand. J. Clin. Lab.
     Invest. 36, 771-777 (1976).

(8) K.D. RAINSFORD. The Effects of Aspirin and other Non-steroid
     Anti-inflammatory/Analgesic Drugs on Gastrointestinal Mucus
     Glycoprotein Biosynthesis In Vivo: Relationship to Ulcero-
     genic Actions. Biochem. Pharmacol. 27, 877-885 (1978).

(9) K.D. RAINSFORD. Electronmicroscopic Observations on the
     Effects of Orally Administered Aspirin and Aspirin-bicarbon-
     ate Mixtures on the Development of Gastric Mucosal Damage in
     the Rat. Gut 16, 514-527 and p. 1001.

(10) J.G. SPENNEY and K.S. MIZE. Inhibition of Gastric K^+ATPase
     by Phenylbutazone and Indomethacin. Biochem. Pharmac. 26,
     1244-1245 (1977).

(11) K.D. LANDECKER, J.E. WELLINGTON, J.H. THOMAS and D.W. PIPER.
     Gastric Ulcer, Aspirin Esterase and Aspirin. In: Aspirin
     and Related Drugs: Their Actions and Uses.
     (Eds. K.D. Rainsford, K. Brune and M.W. Whitehouse).
     Agents and Actions Suppl. 1, 71-79 (1977).

(12) K.D. RAINSFORD and H.M. WATSON. Aspirin Esterase Activity in the Gastric Mucosa of Pigs. Submitted for publication.

(13) K.D. RAINSFORD, N.L.V. FORD, H.M. WATSON and P.M. BROOKS. Aspirin Esterases in Rheumatoid Arthritis and Properties of the Enzymes. Ann. Meeting Aust. Rheumatism Assn. No. 29 (1978).

(14) K.D. RAINSFORD. The Role of Aspirin in Gastric Ulceration. Some Factors Involved in the Development of Gastric Mucosal Damage Induced by Aspirin in Rats Exposed to Various Stress Conditions. Am. J. Dig. Dis. 23, 521-530 (1978).

(15) K.D. RAINSFORD and M.W. WHITEHOUSE. Gastric Irritancy of Aspirin and its Congeners: Anti-inflammatory Activity without this Side-effect. J. Pharm. Pharmac. 28, 599-601 (1976).

(16) R.S. FLOWER. Drugs which Inhibit Prostaglandin Biosynthesis. Pharmac. Revs. 26, 33-67 (1974).

(17) K.D. RAINSFORD. Gastric Mucosal Ulceration Induced by Tablets but not Suspension or Solutions of Aspirin. J. Pharm. Pharmac. 30, 129-131 (1978).

(18) B.J.R. WHITTLE, N.K. BROUGHTON-SMITH, S. MONCADA and J.R. VANE. Actions of Prostacyclin (PGI_2) and its Product, 6-Oxo-PGF_1 on the Rat Gastric Mucosa In Vivo and In Vitro. Prostaglandins 15, 955-967 (1978).

(19) A.K. BANERJEE, J. PHILLIPS and W.M. WINNING. E-type Prostaglandins and Gastric Acid Secretion in the Rat. Nature New Biol. 238, 177-179 (1972).

(20) K. KOWALEWSKI and A. KOLODEJ. Effect of Prostaglandin-E_2 on Gastric Secretion and on Gastric Circulation of Totally Isolated ex vivo Canine Stomach. Pharmacology 11, 85-94 (1974).

(21) S. LINDT and M. BAGGIOLINI. Effect of PG-E_2 Analogue (PG-E_2') on the Vascularization of the Gastric Mucosa in the Rat. Experientia 32, 802 (1976).

(22) K.D. RAINSFORD. On the Cytoprotective Effects of Prostaglandins. In Preparation.

(23) M.M. URSADI, J. FRANCESCHINI and B. MIZZOTTI. Preliminary Investigation on Mast Cell Degranulation and Prostaglandin Involvement in Experimental Gastric Ulceration. Prostaglandins 15, 507-512 (1978).

(24) H.A. CARMICHAEL, L.M. NELSON and R.I. RUSSELL. Cimetidine
     and Prostaglandins: Evidence for Different Modes of Action
     in the Rat Mucosa. Gastroenterology 14, 1229-1232 (1978).

(25) P.H. GUTH, D. AURES and G. PAULSEN. Topical Aspirin Plus HCl
     Gastric Lesions in the Rat. Cytoprotective Effect of Prosta-
     glandin, Cimetidine and Probanthine. Gastroenterology 76,
     88-93 (1979).

(26) K.D. RAINSFORD and M.W. WHITEHOUSE. Gastric Mucus Effusion
     Indicated by Oral Copper Compounds: Potential Anti-Ulcer
     Activity. Experientia 32, 1172-1173 (1976).

(27) A. BENNETT, I.W. STAMFORD and W.G. UNGER. Prostaglandin E_2
     and Gastric Acid Secretion in Man. J. Physiol. 229, 349-
     360 (1973).

(28) C.R. PACE-ASCIAK and G. RANGARAJ. Distribution of Prosta-
     glandin Biosynthetic Pathways in Several Rat Tissues. Forma-
     tion of 6-Ketoprostaglandin $F_{1\alpha}$. Biochim. Biophys. Acta 486,
     579-582 (1977).

(29) H.R. KNAPP, O. OELZ, B.J. SWEETMAN and J.A. OATS. Synthesis
     and Metabolism of Prostaglandins E_2, F_2 and D_2 by the Rat
     Gastrointestinal Tract. Stimulation by Hypertonic Environ-
     ment In Vitro. Prostaglandins 15, 751-757 (1978).

(30) S. MONCADA, J.A. SALMON, J.R. VANE and B.J.R. WHITTLE.
     Formation of Prostacyclin and its Product 6-Oxo-PGF_1 by the
     Gastric Mucosa of Several Species. J. Physiol. 275, 4P-5P.

(31) J.C. MANGLA, Y.M. KIM and A.A. RUBULIS. Aspirin Induced
     Gastric Mucosal Injury in Rats and Adenyl Cyclase. Biochem.
     Med. 11, 376-379 (1974).

(32) J.C. MANGLA, Y.M. KIM and A.A. RUBULS. Adenyl Cyclase Sti-
     mulation by Aspirin in Rat Gastric Mucosa. Nature 250,
     61-62 (1974).

(33) M.S. AMER. Cyclic AMP and Gastric Secretion. Am. J. Dig.
     Dis. 17, 845-849 (1972).

(34) P.R. BIERK, J.A. OATES, G.A. ROBINSON and R.V. ATKINS.
     Cyclic AMP in the Relation of Gastric Secretion in Dogs and
     Humans. Am. J. Physiol. 224, 158-152 (1973).

(35) D.V. KIMBERG. Cyclic Nucleotides and their Role in Gastro-
     intestinal Secretion. Gastroenterology 67, 1032 (1974).

(36) P. MITZNEGG, C.-J. ESTLER, F.W. LOEW and J. van STEL.
     Effects of Salicylates on Cyclic AMP. Hepato-Gastroenterol.
     24, 372-376 (1977).

(37) A.H. SOLL and B.J.R. WHITTLE. Activity of Prostacyclin, a
     stable Analogue, 6B-PGI, and 6-oxo PGF$_1$ on Canine Isolated
     Parietal Cells. Brit. J. Pharmac. 66, 97P-98P (1979).

(38) B. SIMON, H. KATHER and B. KOMMERELL. Effects of Prostaglan-
     dins and their Methylated Analogues upon Human Adenylate
     Cyclase in the Upper Gastro-intestinal Tract. Digestion 17,
     547-553 (1978).

(39) R. ORTMANN and J.P. PERKINS. Stimulation of Adenosine.
     3:5'-Monophosphate Formation by Prostaglandins in Human
     Astrocytoma Cells. Inhibition by Non-steroidal Anti-in-
     flammatory Agents. J. Biol. Chem. 252, 6018-6025 (1977).

(40) G. SACHS, H. CHANG, E. RABON, R. SHACKMAN, H.M. SARAN and
     G. SACCOMAN. Metabolic and Membrane Aspects of Gastric H$^+$
     Transport. Gastroenterology 73, 931-940 (1977).

(41) S.J. HERSEY. Metabolic Changes Associated with Gastric
     Stimulation. Gastroenterology 73, 914-919 (1977).

(42) F.A. KUEHL, J.L. HUMES, G.C. BEVERIDGE, C.G. VAN ARMAN and
     R.W. EGAN. Biologically Active Derivatives of Fatty Acids.
     Prostaglandins, Thromboxanes and Endoperoxides.
     Inflammation 2, 285-294 (1977).

(43) F.A. KUEHL, J.L. HUMES, R.W. EGAN, E.A. HAM, G.C. BEVERIDGE
     and C.G. VAN ARMAN. Role of Prostaglandin Endoperoxide PGG$_2$
     in Inflammatory Processes. Nature 265, 170-173 (1977).

(44) E. EZER, E. PALOSI, G. HAVOS and L. SZPORNY. Antagonism of
     the Gastrointestinal Ulcerogenic Effect of Some Non-steroi-
     dal Anti-inflammatory Agents by Sodium Salicylate.
     J. Pharm. Pharmac. 28, 655-656 (1976).

(45) K.D. RAINSFORD. Comparison of the Ulcerogenic Actions of
     Non-steroid Anti-inflammatory Drugs in Pigs. Agents and
     Actions. Accepted for publication.

(46) Z.N. GAUT, H. BARUTH, L.O. RANDALL, C. AHSLEY and J.R.
     PAULSRUD. Steroisometric Relationship among Anti-inflamma-
     tory Activity. Inhibition of Platelet Aggregation and Inhi-
     bition of Prostaglandin Synthetase. Prostaglandins 10,
     59-66 (1975).

(47) P. KRUPP, R. MENASSE, L. RIESTERER and R. ZIEL. The Biological Significance of Inhibition of Prostaglandin Synthesis. In: The Role of Prostaglandins in Inflammation. (Ed. G.P. Lewis) pp. 106-115, Hans Huber, Berne (1976).

(48) K.D. RAINSFORD. Structure-Activity Relationships of Non-steroid Anti-inflammatory Drugs 1. Gastric Ulcerogenic Activity. Agents and Actions $\underline{8}$, 587-605 (1978).

(49) P. NEEDLEMAN. Experimental Criteria for Evaluating Prostaglandin Biosynthesis and Intrinsic Function. Biochem. Pharmac. $\underline{27}$, 1515-1518 (1978).

(50) R.J. TAYLOR and J.J. SALATA. Inhibition of Prostaglandin Synthetase by Tolmetin (Tolectin, M^{c}N-2559), A New Non-steroidal Anti-inflammatory Agent. Biochem. Pharmac. $\underline{25}$, 2479-2484 (1976).

B.J.R. Whittle

The mechanisms by which aspirin-like compounds damage the gastrointestinal tract has always been a controversial issue. Davenport[1] originally suggested the 'barrier breaking' concept which proposed that aspirin, salicylates as well as bile salts and other such agents, reduced the normal resistance of the gastric mucosa to acid back-diffusion. These agents thus allowed H^+ to diffuse back into the gastric mucosa and hence cause damage. With the finding of Vane[2] that aspirin-like compounds inhibit the biosynthesis of prostaglandins, which were known to occur in, and to have potent actions on the gastric mucosa, an alternative hypothesis was proposed. We suggested that since prostaglandin E_2 was a potent vasodilator in the mucosa, initiation of its formation would lead to a relative fall in mucosal blood flow and hence led to damage and necrosis[3]. More recently we have found prostacyclin (PGI_2) to be the predominant arachidonic acid metabolite in the gastric mucosa, and since it is a more potent vasodilator than PGE_2, it seems likely that prostacyclin and not PGE_2 plays a modulator role in the control of local blood flow[4].

Our studies on the ulcerogenic effects of topical and systemically administered non-steroid anti-inflammatory drugs have thus lead us to the concept of a multi-factorial yet closely linked series of events underlying gastric damage[5]. It is apparent that many aspirin-like compounds have a direct topical irritant action, unrelated to inhibition of prostaglandin biosynthesis. This action shared by surface active agents such as bile salts allows acid to diffuse back into the mucosa as shown originally by Davenport. Although this process leads to gastric damage, the accumulation of H^+ in the mucosa is attenuated by a concurrent rise in local mucosal blood flow. When administered systemically, these aspirin-like agents can also inhibit cyclo-oxygenase, leading to the fall in mucosal blood flow. Such focal areas of ischemia are likely to be the site of damage and erosion formation. It has also been found that systemic cyclo-oxygenase inhibitors greatly enhance the mucosal damage induced by topical irritants. This is presumably the consequence of a reduction in the protective mucosal hyperaemia mentioned above, leading to accumulation of excessive H^+ in the mucosa and hence extensive mucosal damage.

Thus it has become clear that the currently available non-steroid anti-inflammatory compounds can be ranked in order of potency into those which inhibit mucosal cyclo-oxygenase (both when administered systemically or orally) and those which have also a direct topical irritant action. Since both mechanisms interact, the potency of such compounds in producing acute gastric lesions will depend on their relative potency towards both activities. Further studies on the mechanisms underlying those processes and their interaction with other biochemical events occurring simultaneously should help us towards a better understanding of how aspirin-like drugs initiate and promote gastro-intestinal distress.

References

1.   Davenport, H.W. (1964). Gastroenterology, 46, 245-253.

2.   Vane, J.R. (1971). Nature (New Biol.), 231, 232-233.

3.   Main, I.H.M. & Whittle, B.J.R. (1975). Br. J. Pharmacol., 53, 217-224.

4.   Whittle, B.J.R. et al., (1978). Prostaglandins, 15, 955-968.

5.   Whittle, B.J.R. (1977). Br. J. Pharmac., 60, 455-460.

PROSTAGLANDINS AND THE SIDE EFFECTS OF ANTI-INFLAMMATORY DRUGS -
THE KIDNEY.

Keith Crowshaw
May and Baker, Ltd., Dagenham, England.

SUMMARY

        The most important renal side effect of non-steroidal
anti-inflammatory therapy in man is analgesic nephropathy.
One possible mechanism for this effect is inhibition of renal
prostaglandin synthesis. However, an understanding of the
regional biosynthesis of renal prostaglandins, of their pharmacological, physiological and pathological properties in the
kidney and an understanding of the consequences of their inhibition by drugs is required in order to assess whether such a
mechanism is involved.

        These aspects are reviewed, using much of the early
work of the author as a basis for the discussion. The following
conclusions can be drawn from a review of published work. "The
consequences of the inhibition of renal prostaglandin synthesis
do not seem to bear much relationship to the renal side effects
of anti-inflammatory therapy in man". It is further suggested
that impaired renomedullary blood flow arising from decreased
renomedullary PGE_2 synthesis results in increased accumulation
of drug in the renal medulla leading to direct toxic damage.

        Finally, examples of diseases associated with increased
or decreased renal PGE_2 synthesis are discussed and some
examples of drug interactions are presented.

DISCUSSION

        The most important renal side effect of non-steroidal
anti-inflammatory therapy in man is commonly described as
analgesic nephropathy (Table 1).

        The primary event in analgesic nephropathy is ischemic
and toxic damage to intestinal cells, leading initially to renal
papillary necrosis. The subsequent event is intestinal neph-

Table 1   ANALGESIC NEPHROPATHY IN MAN

1. Characterised by: a)   RENAL PAPILLARY NECROSIS
    Followed by: b)   CORTICAL DAMAGE, SCARRING

2. Induced by various non-steroidal anti-inflammatory (N.S.A.I.) agents
    including:

    ASPIRIN   FENOPROFEN

    INDOMETHACIN   ALCLOFENAC

    IBUPROFEN   PHENYLBUTAZONE

3. Lesions are relatively common in patients with rheumatoid arthritis.
        Reference: Prescott (1).

Table 2   SUGGESTED CAUSES OF ANALGESIC NEPHROPATHY

1. Inhibition of renal prostaglandin synthesis

    N.S.A.I. agents can reduce: RENAL BLOOD FLOW

                                   GLOMERULAR FILTRATION RATE

                                   Na^+, H_2O EXCRETION
    leading to MEDULLARY ISCHAEMIA and ATROPHY.

2. Chronic renal tubular injury
    Leading to ATROPHIC PAPILLARY NECROSIS,
    caused by ACETYLATION OF TUBULAR CELL PROTEINS (only applicable to
    aspirin, phenacetin, paracetamol).

3. Inhibition of renal phosphodiesterase
    (Indomethacin, others?).

itis, which is a non-specific cortical change caused by obstruction of tubules in the renal medulla.

The worst examples of analgesic nephropathy are seen in patients who abuse analgesic preparations containing combinations of aspirin, paracetamol and phenacetin. Data provided by the Committee on Safety of Medicines for the period March 1964 to December 1975 (2) suggests that the therapeutic use of a number of different non-steroidal anti-inflammatory agents can be correlated with adverse renal reactions albeit in relatively few numbers of patients.

Toxicological data in animals, most commonly rats, also confirms that aspirin is a more potent inducer of nephropathy when administered together with paracetamol or phenacetin than it is when administered alone (3). In this paper Nanra and co-workers review the data obtained from patients treated with large doses of aspirin over many years. In patients taking aspirin for chronic rheumatoid arthritis they discuss several references which demonstrate that at autopsy or biopsy, the incidence of renal papillary necrosis and chronic intestinal nephritis is high (it varies from 8 to 100%). However, these renal lesions, although identical to those seen in analgesic nephropathy, are less severe and these patients rarely present with severe renal failure.

Non-steroidal anti-inflammatory agents have numerous properties which could cause nephropathy (Table 2). The first of these listed in Table 2 shows the main topic of this paper. However, I would emphasise that inhibition of renal prostaglandin synthesis is only one of a large number of possible mechanisms which could be involved in causing analgesic nephropathy. For example during the concentration of urine in the kidney, particularly in the renal medulla, large concentrations of drug or its metabolites can be present in the nephrons and blood vessels and this may lead to direct toxic effects. In the case of aspirin these toxic effects could be caused by acetylation of renal enzymes although there are in addition other potential biochemical mechanisms which could be involved. Aspirin or salicylate, for example, are known to interfere with the tri-carboxylic cycle, with oxidative phosphorylation and with mucopolysaccaride synthesis and paracetamol and phenacetin can cause oxidative changes leading to glucose-6-phosphate dehydro-genase, glutathione and NADPH deficiencies. Another possibility suggested is an interference with cyclic AMP dependent renal mechanisms through inhibition of phosphodiesterases by drugs such as indomethacin. However, there is no data which indicates that this property could lead directly to toxic effects.

This paper discusses the evidence suggesting that inhibition of renal prostaglandin synthetase is a potential

cause of nephropathy.   However, in order to do this, it is
necessary to know which prostaglandins are present in the renal
medulla and cortex, and to assess the physiological and pathological actions of these prostaglandins in the kidney.   Only
then is it possible to assess the possible consequences of
inhibition of these compounds by non-steroidal anti-inflammatory
agents.

        Very little work has been done on human kidney, most
studies having been performed in the rabbit, rat or dog.   In
1974 Crowshaw and McGiff reviewed this evidence correlating the
biochemical formation and metabolism of the renal prostaglandins
with their possible renal functions (4,5).   At that time it was
known that only the renal cortex contained an active metabolising
enzyme system for the inactivation of PGE_2 and $PGF_{2\alpha}$, the
activity being low in the renal medulla.   In addition the only
two renal prostaglandins identified in the kidney of dogs and
rabbits were PGE_2 and $PGF_{2\alpha}$, located almost exclusively in the
renal medulla.   However, as analytical techniques improved it
became apparent that the renal cortex is also capable of
synthesising both PGE_2 and $PGF_{2\alpha}$ (Table 3).   However, this
relatively simple view of the distribution of prostaglandins
in kidney has become more confused by the recent discoveries of
thromboxanes and prostacyclin.   Morrison et al (7) reported
that uretal obstruction in rabbit kidney for three days induces
the ability to generate TXA_2 following stimulation by bradykinin
infusion.   The uretal obstructed kidney could also generate
TXA_2 *in vitro*, in contrast to the contralateral 'normal' kidney
which only synthesised the prostaglandins shown in Table 3.
Oates and his group (8) have also demonstrated synthesis of
prostacyclin by rabbit renal cortex microsomes (Table 4).

        Recent work (reviewed by Bolger (9)) indicates that
both PGE_2 and PGI_2 stimulated the release of renin from the
renal cortex and it has been suggested that $PGF_{2\alpha}$ may inhibit
renin release.   Thus the finding that both $PGF_{2\alpha}$ and PGI_2 can
be synthesised in the renal cortex (Table 4) suggests that
these prostaglandins could modulate renin release depending on
the predominant cortical prostaglandin or prostacyclin release.

        Likewise earlier work by Lonigro (10) demonstrated a
clear dependency of renal blood flow on synthesis of PGE_2,
presumably by the renal medulla, in anaesthetised dogs.   This
work was confirmed by other workers and an excellent discussion
of the role of prostaglandins in renal function can be found in
the review by Flamenbaum and Kleinmann (11).   However, Zins
(12) did not observe any alteration in renal blood flow after
the administration of indomethacin to unanaesthetised dogs.
This result suggests that the activation of the sympathetic
nervous system, as well as the renin-angiotensin system, by
anaesthetics resulted in the stimulation of PGE_2 release from
the kidney, thus increasing the renal blood flow well above
normal resting levels.   Since there are a number of well

Table 3   DISTRIBUTION OF PROSTAGLANDINS IN THE RABBIT KIDNEY

Prostaglandins generated in homogenates of rabbit renal cortex and medulla were estimated by a mass spectrometric method.

	Cortex µg/g	Medulla µg/g
PGE_2	0.19	4.36
$PGF_{2\alpha}$	0.21	1.64
PGA_2	0.015*	0.21*

* Not corrected for the observed 8% conversion of tracer PGE_2 to PGA_2 during the experiment.

C. Larsson and E. Anggard, 1976 (6).

Table 4   REGIONAL DIFFERENCES IN PROSTACYCLIN
               FORMATION BY RABBIT KIDNEY

Estimates of PGI_2 and other PGs synthesised in microsomes of renal cortex and medulla using PGG_2 or arachidonic acid as substrate were obtained.   Mass spectral confirmation for the identification of 6-keto-$PGF_{1\alpha}$ was also obtained.

	Percent conversion	
	Cortex	Medulla
PGE_2	14.8	92.9
$PGF_{2\alpha}$	60.5	6.0
PGD_2	6.9	1.0
6-keto-$PGF_{1\alpha}$	17.8	N.D.

Whorton et al, 1978 (8).

documented vasoconstrictor interventions which can release renal PGE_2, namely renal artery constriction, renal nerve stimulation, noradrenaline infusion and angiotensin infusion (13), it is a reasonable hypothesis that the renal medulla releases vasodilator PGE_2 in response to vasoconstrictor influences as a defensive mechanism.

CONCLUSIONS

Possible physiological functions of the renal prostaglandins

1.   Renal PGE_2 and prostacyclin are unlikely to be important for maintenance of renal blood flow under normal resting conditions.

2.   They are probably important for the maintenance of blood flow when it is reduced in

   a)   Circulatory failure
   b)   Dehydration
   c)   Renal artery disease
   d)   Under conditions of hormonal or nerve-mediated renal vasoconstriction.

3.   They are probably important in Na^+, K^+ and water homeostasis, and in the regulation of renin release from the kidney.

Additional circumstantial evidence in support of these possible mechanisms can be derived from the observed clinical effects of indomethacin in man (Table 5).

The consequences of inhibition of renal prostaglandin synthesis do not seem to bear much relationship to the renal side effects of anti-inflammatory therapy in man as discussed earlier in this paper. On the basis of present evidence, it is not justifiable to state with any certainty that such side effects can be attributed to the inhibition of prostaglandin synthesis.

However, it is the opinion of the author that decreased renomedullary PGE_2 synthesis results in the kidney being deprived of one of its primary vasodilator defensive mechanisms which normally acts to oppose the effects of endogenous vaso-constrictor agents in the kidney. Since the released PGE_2 can only be a vasodilator in the renal medulla, then its inhibition by non-steroidal anti-inflammatory agents will result in an enhanced constrictor response to other vasoconstrictor mechanisms arising from pre-existing conditions in certain patients, e.g. renal artery disease, hypotension, increased activity of the renin-angiotensin system, catecholamine secreting tumors, etc.. One consequence arising from decreased

Table 5   PHARMACOLOGICAL EFFECTS OF N.S.A.I. AGENTS
                        ON RENAL FUNCTION IN MAN

        1.   Increased blood pressure

        2.   Decreased renal blood flow

        3.   Decreased renin release

        4.   Decreased plasma aldosterone

        5.   Decreased Na^+ excretion

        6.   Decreased urinary PGE_2

       References (14, 15, 16)

Table 6   CLINICAL CONDITIONS AFFECTED BY RENAL
            PROSTAGLANDIN PRODUCTION AND N.S.A.I. AGENTS

	Clinical diagnosis	Characteristics	Effect of N.S.A.I. therapy
1.	BARTTER'S SYNDROME	↑Renin	↓Renin
		↑Aldosterone	↓Aldosterone
		↑K^+ excretion	↓K^+ exretion
		↑PGE_2 synthesis	↓PGE_2 synthesis
		Juxtaglomerular hyperplasia	–
		Normal b.p.	B.p. unchanged
2.	LUPUS ERYTHEMATOSUS	Nephritis	
		Renal inflammation	↓Renal function
		↑PGE_2 synthesis	↓PGE_2 synthesis
3.	HYPORENINAEMIA	↓Renin	
	HYPOALDOSTERONISM	↓Aldosterone	
		↓K^+ excretion	*
		↓PGE synthesis	

* Contra-indicated – however in a patient with mild renal failure, indomethacin induced identical symptoms (18, 19).

Table 7   MODIFICATION OF DRUG ACTION BY N.S.A.I. AGENTS

Drug	Therapeutic effect	Effect of N.S.A.I. therapy
Furosemide* (Ref.19)	Antihypertensive diuretic	Reverses Diuresis
	$\uparrow$Renal blood flow	$\downarrow$Na$^+$ excretion
	$\uparrow$Renin	$\downarrow$Renin
Spironolactone (Ref.20,21)	Natriuretic	Antagonised by aspirin
	$\uparrow$Renal PGE$_2$ synthesis	$\downarrow$PGE$_2$ synthesis
Clonidine (Ref.23,24)	Antihypertensive (a-adrenergic agent)	
	Diuretic	Antagonised by indo- methacin
	$\uparrow$Renal PGE$_2$ synthesis	$\downarrow$PGE$_2$ synthesis

* The diuretic action of hydrochlorthiazide is not modified by indomethacin.

renomedullary blood flow is that there is likely to be an accumulation of drug or its metabolites in the renal medulla, and this increased accumulation of drug could result in direct toxic damage to the renal medulla, as seen in analgesic nephropathy for example.   The author is not aware of any direct evidence to support this hypothesis.   However, the data that could eventually confirm this hypothesis will come from clinical observations of diseases which arise from an excess (Bartter's syndrome and lupus erythematosus) or a deficiency of renal prostaglandin production (hypereninaemia and hyper-aldosteronism) and it would be of interest to know if patients with the latter condition develop the same renal side effects as those patients on high doses of aspirin.

Finally an unusual but potentially important example of the side effects of non-steroidal anti-inflammatory therapy is shown in Table 7.   It is now becoming apparent that a number of drugs which have their primary site of action in the kidney act at least in part by mechanisms which increase the renal concentration of PGE_2.   For example it has been suggested that furosemide inhibits 15-hydroxy prostaglandin dehydrogenase and spirinolactone and clonidine have been shown to stimulate PGE_2 synthesis.   The administration of prostaglandin synthetase inhibitors to patients already receiving any of these drugs could affect the therapeutic effectiveness of these latter agents, with potential serious consequences.

REFERENCES

(1)   PRESCOTT,L.F.   The nephrotoxicity and hepatotoxicity of antipyretic analgesics.   Brit.J.Clin.Pharmac., 7, 453-462 (1979).

(2)   SHELLEY,J.H.   Pharmacological mechanisms of analgesic nephropathy.   Kidney International, 13, 15-26 (1978).

(3)   NANRA,R.S., STUART-TAYLOR,J., DE LEON,A.H. and WHITE, K.H.   Analgesic nephropathy: etiology, clinical syndrome and clinicopathologic correlations in Australia.   Kidney International, 13, 79-92 (1978).

(4)   CROWSHAW,K. and McGIFF,J.C. in "Proceedings, International workshop conference on mechanisms of hypotension", ed. Sambti,H.P.   Excerpta Medical Foundation, 254-273 (1974).

(5)   McGIFF,J.C., CROWSHAW,K. and ITSKOVITZ,H.D.   Prostaglandins and renal function.   Fed.Proc., 33, 39-47 (1974).

(6)   LARSSON,C. and ANGGARD,E.   Mass spectrometric determination of prostaglandin E_2, $F_{2\alpha}$ and A_2 in the cortex

and medulla of the rabbit kidney.   J.Pharm.Pharmacol.,
28, 326-327 (1976).

(7)   MORRISON,A.R., NISHIKAWA,K. and NEEDLEMAN,P.   Un-
masking of thromboxane A_2 synthesis by ureteral
obstruction in the rabbit kidney.   Nature, 267,
259-260 (1977).

(8)   WHORTON,A.R., SMIGEL,H., OATES,J.A. and FROLICH,J.C.
Regional differences in prostacyclin formation by the
kidney.   Prostacyclin is a major prostaglandin of
renal cortex.   Biochem.Biophys.Acta, 529, 176-180
(1978).

(9)   BOLGER,P.M., EISNER,G.H., RAMWELL,P.W., SLOTTCOFF,L.M.
and COREY,E.J.   Renal actions of prostacyclin.
Nature, 271, 467-469 (1978).

(10)   LONIGRO,A.J., ITSKOVITZ,H.D., CROWSHAW,K. and McGIFF,
J.C.   Dependency of renal blood flow on prostaglandin
synthesis in the dog.   Circulation Research, 32,
712-717 (1973).

(11)   FLAMENBAUM,W.F. and KLEINMAN,J.G. in "The Prostaglandins", volume 3, ed. Ramwell,P.W., Plenum Press,
London, 267-328 (1977).

(12)   ZINS,G.R.   Renal prostaglandins.   Am.J.Med., 58,
14-24 (1975).

(13)   McGIFF,J.C., CROWSHAW,K., TERRAGNO,N.A. and LUNIGRO,
A.J.   Renal prostaglandins: possible regulators of
the renal actions of pressor hormones.   Nature, 227,
1255-1257 (1970).

(14)   FROLICH,J.C., in "The Prostaglandins", volume 3,
ed. Ramwell,P.W., Plenum Press, London, 1-39 (1977).

(15)   BRATES,D.C., ANDERSON,S.A. and STRONIG,S.   Azosemide,
a "loop" diuretic and furosemide.   Clin.Pharmacol.
Ther., 25, 322-330 (1979).

(16)   RANE,A., OELZ,O., FROLICH,J.C., SEYBERTH,K.W., SWEET-
MAN, B.J., WATSON,J.T., WILKINSON,G.R. and OATES,J.A.
Relation between plasma concentration of indomethacin
and its effects on prostaglandin synthesis and platelet
aggregation in man.   Clin.Pharmacol.Ther., 23, 658-
668 (1978).

(17)   NORBY,L.H., WEIDIG,J., RAMWELL,P., SLOTKOFF,L. and
FLAMENBAUM,W.   Possible role for impaired renal
prostaglandin production in the pathogenesis of hypo-
reninaemia.   Lancet,2, 1118-1122 (1978).

(18)   TAN,S.Y., SHAPIRO,R. and MULROW,P.J.   Renal prosta-
        glandins exert major influence on the renin-aldo-
        sterone axis and on K⁺ hemostasis.   Clin.Res., 25,
        598A (1977).

(19)   OLIW,E., KÖVÉR,G. and LARSSON,C.   Reduction by indo-
        methacin of furosemide effects in the rabbit.   Europ.
        J.Pharmacol., 38, 95-100 (1976).

(20)   TWEEDALE,M.G. and OGILVIE,R.I.   Antagonism of
        spinnolactone-induced natriuresis by aspirin in man.
        Europ.J.Pharmacol., 38, 95-100 (1976).

(21)   PAPANICOLAOU,N., McNEIL,B.J., FUNKENSTEIN,H.H. and
        SUDARSKY,L.R.   Interaction between aldosterone and
        renomedullary prostaglandins.   Competitive action
        between aspirin and spinnolactone.   Experentia, 33,
        1632-1634 (1977).

(22)   OLSEN,U.B.   Clonidine-induced increase of renal
        prostaglandin activity and water diuresis in the dog.
        Europ.J.Pharmacol., 36, 95-101 (1976).

(23)   ERCAN,Z.S., BOR,N.M. and TURKER,R.K.   The role of
        endogenous prostaglandins in the renal response to
        clonidine.   Arch.Int.Pharmacodyn., 239, 319-325 (1979).

SUMMING UP

G. P. Lewis

One of the most important recent advances is the discovery of more and more products of arachidonic acid metabolism. Clearly there are going to be great developments in elucidating the role played by the products of the lipoxygenase pathways, not only in those related to SRS-A, but in mechanisms which might involve a switching of metabolism of arachidonic acid from the cyclo-oxygenase to the lipoxygenase pathways. There appears to be some evidence that arachidonic acid metabolites other than PGs might even be involved in temperature control.

It seems likely that products of lipoxygenase might play a role in chemotaxis and in some concentrations inhibitors of cyclo-oxygenase might well increase some inflammatory effects such as the migration of cells, by diverting arachidonic acid metabolism to hydroxy acids.

One factor which might well be important in chronic inflammation is that some PGs produce an anti-granuloma effect possibly via stimulation of cAMP. However, the conditions under which this effect occurs are not at all clear. When we came to consider the role of PGs in the regulation of cellular activities we were presented with some strong views although not always backed up by experimental evidence. It seems that PGs play little part in the activity of polymorphonuclear leucocytes. These cells release a battery of enzymes and it was suggested that any factors released which might activate the PG system are incidental.

Macrophages present a different picture however. We now know that activated macrophages produce a series of PGs - E_2, I_2 (or its metabolite) TxB_2 and $PGF_2\alpha$. Furthermore there is evidence from several workers that PGs inhibit lymphocyte function and the view still holds that a negative

feed-back mechanism for macrophage-PGs regulating lymphocyte
activities might be a natural mechanism.   However, once again
the warning came through that several other factors produced
by macrophages influence the activities of other cells
including lymphocytes either causing activation or inhibition.
The view that RA patients possess lymphocytes which have a
lower than normal sensitivity to PGs has not yet received any
experimental support.

One of the most important questions I asked in the
introduction of the Symposium was, are we sure that the anti-
inflammatory activity of non-steroid anti-inflammatory drugs
is due to their inhibition of PG synthesis.   I suggested
that we should limit this statement to vascular and analgesic
effects, and although there were one or two doubters, I should
say that there is general agreement that the relief of pain
and swelling by anti-inflammatory drugs can be largely
accounted for in this way.   On the other hand, there is also
agreement that these agents have effects other than inhibiting
cyclo-oxygenase.

When considering correlations between clinical
efficacy and enzyme inhibition, we must take into account not
only the test system used but bio availability, metabolism
and other factors.   However, it was pointed out clearly that
within a limited group of anti-inflammatory agents, where
these variables were controlled, one could obtain good
correlation between biological activity and inhibition of PG
synthesis.

On the question of specificity of various tissue
cyclo-oxygenases, there does seem to be some evidence that
differences exist.   Most recently aspirin has been shown
to be more active against platelet cyclo-oxygenase than that
in some other cells.   Furthermore it has been suggested that
there are certain compounds which protect against the gastro-
intestinal irritation but do not interfere with their anti-
inflammatory activity.   This might also be interpreted as a
differential activity of the drugs on the different cyclo-
oxygenases.

Non-steroid anti-inflammatory agents have a lot of side-effects although gastro-intestinal irritation is probably the most common. Prostaglandins inhibit acid secretion, probably regulate blood flow, cause mucous secretion and maybe have a cytoprotective action. Removal of these PG-mediated effects by cyclo-oxygenase inhibitors, strongly indicates that part of their toxicity is due to inhibition of PG synthesis. Some correlation has been shown between anti-oedema activity and gastric ulcer activity. However, once again it was emphasised that some of the agents have additional properties which might differ from one to the other and these factors must be taken into account in trying to show correlations of activities. Furthermore, we hear that there is the possibility of direct damage after oral administration as well as that due to inhibition of cyclo-oxygenase. In addition, since these acids are absorbed through the gastric mucosa to a large extent, the tissue is more likely to suffer from their damaging effects.

With toxic effects in the kidney, the story appears to be the same - some of the effects are due to inhibition of PG synthesis, but as these agents exert several other biochemical effects, these might also be important in producing their toxic side-effects.

We have not heard much about the possible role of thromboxane in inflammation, but perhaps this is because of the difficulty of its determination. Now that we are learning about new metabolites which are different from TxB_2, perhaps this will give us additional tools to analyse this part of the arachidonic acid pathway.

It is not always possible to assess immediately the value of a meeting such as we have had during the last two days. Sometimes we need to digest the new information to which we have been exposed before reaping the benefit. However, one can get a good idea of the success of a meeting by the interest and participation of the audience. There is no doubt that we have had a full participation here. The discussions after each section have been interesting and relevant. We must thank our hosts for choosing such a well-balanced programme.

SUBJECT INDEX